# Manipal Manual of

# Endoscopic Sinus Surgery

## Second Edition

# Manipal Manual of
# Endoscopic Sinus Surgery

## Second Edition

### Dipak Ranjan Nayak
MBBD, MS, FICS, Fellow of UICC

Professor and Head
Department of ENT–Head & Neck Surgery
Kasturba Medical College
Manipal

### Produl Hazarika
MBBS, DLO, MS, FACS, FRCS (Edin), FIAO FUWAI, Fellow of UICC

Ex-Professor and Head
Department of ENT–Head & Neck Surgery
Kasturba Medical College
Manipal

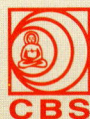

# CBS Publishers & Distributors Pvt Ltd

New Delhi • Bengaluru • Chennai • Kochi • Pune
Hyderabad • Kolkata • Mumbai • Nagpur • Patna

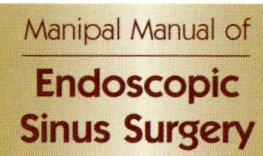

Manipal Manual of
**Endoscopic Sinus Surgery**

ISBN: 978-81-239-2292-8

Copyright © Authors and Publisher

**Second Edition:** 2013

First Edition: 2008

Published by Satish Kumar Jain for

**CBS Publishers & Distributors** Pvt Ltd
*Head Office:* 4819/XI Prahlad Street, 24 Ansari Road, Daryaganj, New Delhi 110 002, India.
Ph: 23289259, 23266861, 23266867       Fax: 011-23243014       e-mail: delhi@cbspd.com; cbspubs@airtelmail.in       Website: www.cbspd.com

*Corporate Office:* 204 FIE, Industrial Area, Patparganj, Delhi 110 092
Ph: 4934 4934                Fax: 4934 4935            e-mail: publishing@cbspd.com; publicity@cbspd.com

*Branches*

- **Bengaluru:** Seema House 2975, 17th Cross, K.R. Road,
  Banasankari 2nd Stage, Bengaluru 560 070, Karnataka
  Ph: +91-80-26771678/79            Fax: +91-80-26771680         e-mail: bangalore@cbspd.com
- **Chennai:** 20, West Park Road, Shenoy Nagar, Chennai 600 030, Tamil Nadu
  Ph: +91-44-26260666, 26208620        Fax: +91-44-42032115       e-mail: chennai@cbspd.com
- **Kochi:** 36/14 Kalluvilakam, Lissie Hospital Road, Kochi 682 018, Kerala
  Ph: +91-484-4059061-65            Fax: +91-484-4059065        e-mail: kochi@cbspd.com
- **Pune:** Bhuruk Prestige, Sr. No. 52/12/2+1+3/2 Narhe, Haveli
  (Near Katraj-Dehu Road Bypass), Pune 411 041, Maharashtra
  Ph: +91-20-64704058, 64704059, 32392277        Fax: +91-20-24300160       e-mail: pune@cbspd.com

*Representatives*

- **Hyderabad**   0-9885175004      • **Kolkata**   0-9831437309, 0-9051152362      • **Mumbai**   0-9833017933
- **Nagpur**   0-9021734563      • **Patna**   0-9334159340

*Printed at* Magic International Pvt Ltd, Greater Noida, UP

# Foreword

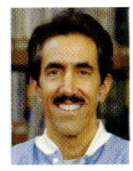

Contemporary rhinology is currently an "unsettled" discipline with two distinct philosophical camps. The origin of this rift begins with the introduction of the "functional" concept of sinus surgery by Messerklinger in 1978. He proposed that "surgery on the sinus prechambers" would eliminate the need for surgery on the sinuses themselves, and that mucociliary clearance was the crucial element of sinus physiology. Ironically, the maxillary antrostomy was never conceived or envisioned by Messerklinger, and never described in his "functional thesis", yet became the hallmark of FESS.

In the mid-1990's, true minimally invasive sinus procedures were conceived and introduced by Setliff and Nayak. These procedures more closely followed the teachings of Messerklinger by introducing a stepwise approach to sinus surgery based on specific anatomic landmarks and eliminating the maxillary antrostomy from the procedure, and even preserving the uncinate process. Outcomes from these procedures have been shown to exceed those from conventional FESS across the spectrum of disease, while also reducing operative time, surgical morbidity, and recovery time for patients. However, these advances were originally met with significant resistance by the majority of rhinologists who refused to question the necessity of the antrostomy—a procedure that has never been shown to be necessary or even beneficial by any clinical trial.

Since the advent of limited targeted surgery, the minimally invasive movement has gained in popularity among surgeons and patients. Newer technologies, such as balloon sinuplasty, continue to challenge our understanding of sinus physiology by providing even less invasive options for sinus sufferers. However, despite these significant advances of the minimally invasive "movement", many rhinologists fail to embrace this mounting body of evidence. The authors of *Manipal Manual of Endoscopic Sinus Surgery* share the vision of minimally invasive rhinology and have dedicated this text to further advancing our knowledge in the field. Their pioneering work is to be applauded as it raises the standard of sinus care for all.

**Peter Catalano** MD, FACS, FARS

Chief of Otolaryngology
St. Elizabeth's Medical Center
Professor of Otolaryngology
Tufts University School of Medicine
Boston, Massachusetts, USA

# Preface to the Second Edition

It is a great pleasure to bring out the second edition of the *Manipal Manual of Endoscopic Sinus Surgery*. The first edition of this picturesque atlas received overwhelming response, suggestions and criticism. Most of the queries have been addressed to satisfy the readers. In the second edition, four new chapters have been added including chapters on balloon sinuplasty, CSF rhinorrhea, and allergic fungal rhinosinusitis written by the first author (DRN). New photographs and illustrations have been added from the personal album of DRN. The fourth new chapter has been written by our guest author from Malaysia, Dr Jaspal Singh Sahota, on "The role of nasal endoscopy on nasopharyngeal cancer". Dr Peter Catalano has written the Foreword to the second edition. We sincerely hope this edition will be an encouraging force for the beginners and the postgraduates to learn and practise the art of endoscopic sinus surgery, the concept of which was developed by Messerklinger and popularized and developed further by Stammberger, Kenedy and Draf.

**Dipak Ranjan Nayak**
**Produl Hazarika**

# Preface to the First Edition

Functional endoscopic sinus surgery has now been well accepted as a standard treatment modality for chronic sinusitis. Since its introduction by Messerklinger in 1978, there was some resistance from many rhinologists to accept this technique as a modality of treatment for chronic sinusitis. With persistent effort from his student Stammberger and later David Kennedy to convince the rest of the world regarding its efficacy through proper documentation, it has now been the most popular and accepted modality of treatment for chronic sinusitis. The failure of endoscopic sinus surgery does not pertain to the nasal condition or disease but is due to the inability of the surgeon to understand the intricate and complex anatomy and physiology of ostiomeatal complex that can be achieved by extensive theoretical and practical knowledge through laboratory studies and cadaveric dissection.

This book is aimed at particularly the beginners in the field of endoscopic sinus surgery to provide adequate knowledge of microanatomy and physiology of the nose and paranasal sinuses, the pathophysiology of chronic sinusitis and related diseases and a systematic endoscopic approach to manage such conditions effectively. A number of colour photographs and drawings have been incorporated to make the book in colour atlas format for easy understanding by the reader.

Dipak Ranjan Nayak
Produl Hazarika

# Acknowledgements

It is now and only after completion of our work that we realize the immense necessity of writing this page in an effort to acknowledge those who in all their possible ways have helped us in carrying out and completing the second edition of the book.

We take the privilege to express our profound sense of gratitude to our teachers late Prof BR Das of Assam and Prof MC Sahoo and Prof G Behera of Cuttack for their influence in initiating this project of ours. We have the pleasure to place on record the concise and concrete suggestions as well as the goodwill offered to us by Prof LH Hiranandani, Prof K Kameshwaran, Prof AL Mukherjee, Prof KK Ramlingam, Prof RC Deka, Dr Vishanathan, Dr Mahadeviah and Dr Mohan Kameswaran. We owe a deep sense of gratitude to these great teachers of otolaryngology of our time.

We deeply appreciate and thank Dr Peter Catalano, St. Elizabeth's Medical Center, USA, for writing the Foreword to the second edition of this book.

Our special thanks to Prof Santosh Kackar, former Professor of ENT and Director, All India Institute of Medical Sciences, New Delhi, for writing the Foreword to the first edition.

We are grateful to our founder beloved President of MAHE, Dr Ram Das M Pai; Dr HS Ballal, Pro Chancellor of Manipal University; and Dr S Rao, Dean of KMC, Manipal, who have kindly permitted us to complete the work on this book, lacking which, we fear, it would not have been possible to bring this work to light.

It is worthwhile to express a word of appreciation to Dr Suresh Pillai, Dr Sherry Jacob, Dr Kailesh Pujary, Dr Parul Pujary, Dr Asha Kumar, Dr Sajeev George, Dr SA Mallik, Dr Vivek, C Abraham, Dr NLN Reddy, Dr A Suneel, Dr Navneet, Dr Avneesh, Dr Ajay Lavania, Dr Raghavendra Rao, Dr Ramananda Shetty, Dr Rodney Rodrigues, Dr Hemant, Dr Harish Kundaje, Dr Mahesh, Dr Ranveer, Dr Seema EP, Dr Pallavi, Dr Sunil, Dr Deepika, Dr Sajilal, Dr Aishwarya, Dr Vijaya, Dr Ramakrishna, Dr Deepa, Dr Archana, Dr Jyothi, Dr Gopi, Dr Abhishek, Dr Deichu, Dr Navneeta, Dr Ajay, Dr Ashish, Dr Kumar Raja, Dr Nadia, Dr Sandeep, Dr Harish, Dr Shruti and Dr Susan.

Special thanks to Dr Sandeep (Sr) Harshita, Dr Keshav and Dr Manu for helping us in proofreading of the second edition.

We also deeply appreciate Dr Balakrishna, Professor, ENT, and Dr Rohit Singh, Assistant Professor, ENT, for contributing to Chapters 6 and 12 in the first edition of this book and Dr Jaspal Singh Sahota for Chapter 18 in the second edition.

We shall be failing in our duties if we do not offer our heartful gratitude to our parents late Mr and Mrs LC Hazarika and late Mrs and Dr B Nayak, Prof KR Iyengar and Mrs Lakshmi Iyengar. We are also thankful to our wives and children Miss Sweta and Master Sundeep Nayak, Dr Manali Hazarika, and Mrinmoy Hazarika, for their constant encouragement and support.

Our secretary Mrs Latha also deserves our thanks for help along with nonteaching staff of the Department Mr Seetharam, Mrs Mangala, Mr Bhaskar, Mr Sudhakar, and Sister (Mrs) Shanthi, Mrs Malathi, Mrs Mohini, Mrs Usha, Mrs Baby, Mrs Vasanthi and Mrs Bhavani.

We offer our gratefulness to our patients who so optimistically offer themselves to our surgical efforts to cure such diseases.

**Dipak Ranjan Nayak | Produl Hazarika**

# Contents

# Anatomical Considerations— Nose and PNS

A precise knowledge of the anatomy of the nasal cavity and the paranasal sinuses, especially that of the lateral wall of the nose, the sphenoethmo-frontal sinuses and their relation to the adjacent vital structures, is essential to understand the pathophysiology and management of chronic sinusitis and is mandatory before venturing on an effective and safe endoscopic sinus surgery. Vital structures like the orbit, cranial cavity, optic nerve, internal carotid artery, etc. lie in close relation to the sphenoethmofrontal sinuses, usually separated by a thin bone; making them vulnerable to injury during an endoscopic sinus surgery.

The exact orientation of various intranasal and extranasal structures regarding their location, attitude and interrelation can be studied only by repeated cadaveric dissections. Knowledge of these and that of their variations is useful in diagnostics and invaluable in surgery and endoscopic approaches that have gained popularity for septoplasty, septorhinoplasty, adenoidectomy, hypophysectomy, excision of benign tumors like angiofibroma, inverted papilloma, glioma, etc.

The introduction of nasal and sinus endoscopy, better imaging techniques and study of whole organ mounted sections has helped us to understand better the micro architectural anatomy of sphenoethmoids and their vital relations.

## SKELETAL FRAMEWORK OF EXTERNAL NOSE
(Fig. 1.1)

It consists of bony and cartilaginous supportive framework.

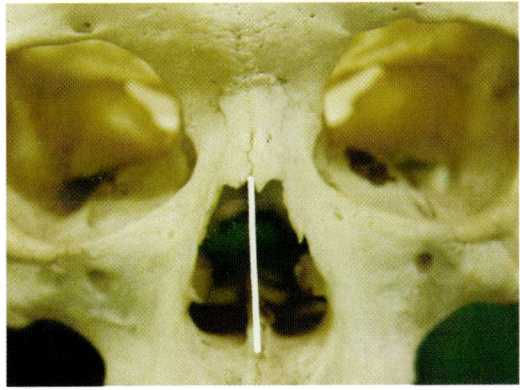

**Fig. 1.1:** Bony skeletal framework of external nose and orbit

**Bony part consists of the following** (Fig. 1.2)
1. Paired nasal bone
2. Paired frontal process of the maxilla
3. Nasal process of the frontal bone.

Nasal bone articulates with the nasal process of the frontal bone superiorly, frontal process of the maxilla laterally, inferiorly with the upper lateral cartilage and medially with nasal bone of the other side. The junction between the two nasal bones forms the bridge of the nose. The nasal bone ossifies in membrane from one center overlying the anterior part of the cartilaginous nasal capsule.

## Cartilaginous part is made up of the following cartilages

1. Paired upper lateral cartilage.
2. Paired lower lateral cartilage (alar cartilages)

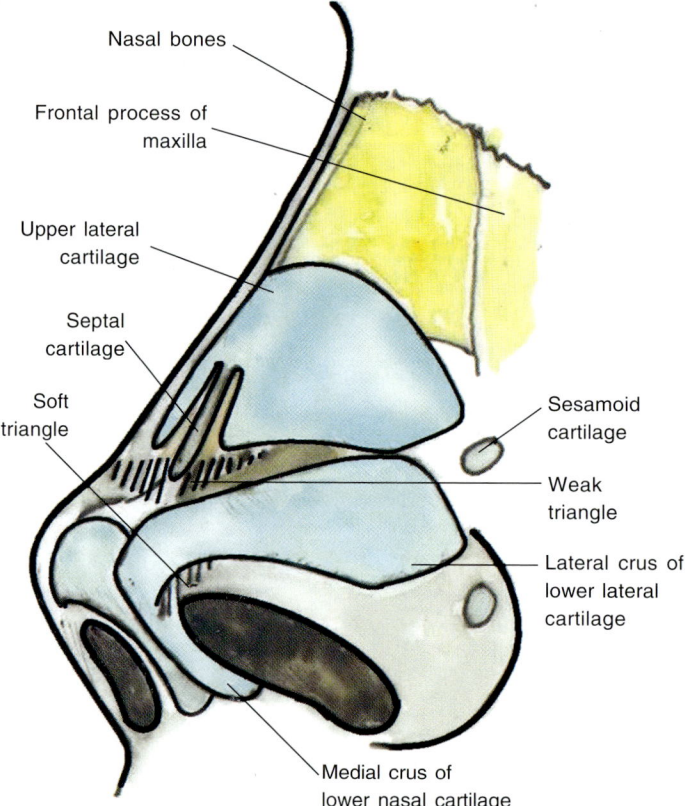

**Fig. 1.2:** Skeletal framework of external nose

Labels: Nasal bones, Frontal process of maxilla, Upper lateral cartilage, Septal cartilage, Soft triangle, Sesamoid cartilage, Weak triangle, Lateral crus of lower lateral cartilage, Medial crus of lower nasal cartilage

3. Sesamoid cartilage
4. Anterior part of the septal cartilage.

The upper lateral cartilage is triangular in shape and is attached above with the frontal process of maxilla and inferior margin of nasal bone. Medially it is continuous with the septal cartilage and in fact is a triangular flat expansion of the septal cartilage forming the middle third of the nose.

**The lower lateral cartilage** or the alar cartilage forms the lower third of the nose and is responsible for maintaining the projection and shape of the tip. It consists of slender medial crus and wider lateral crus. The two medial crurae support the columella. Each lateral crus forms the ala of the nose. The projection between the medial and lateral crurae of the cartilage supports the tip of the nose, that forms the dome.

The minor sesamoid cartilages are present between the upper and lower nasal cartilages.

The nasal cartilages are made up of hyaline cartilage. Nasal bones and cartilages are connected to each other by periosteum and perichondrium, which is continuous. The upper and lower lateral cartilages prevent collapse of the vestibule during inspiration.

The skin covers the skeletal framework of the external nose, which is continuous with the skin of the columella and vestibule of the nose.

## NASAL CAVITY

The nasal cavity is divided into right and left nasal cavities by the nasal septum. Each nasal cavity has a medial and a lateral wall, a roof and a floor. The anterior most part of the nasal cavities lined by the skin is called the vestibule of the nose. Rest of the nasal cavities is lined by the respiratory epithelium below and olfactory epithelium above (dangerous area of nose). Each nasal cavity is approximately 5–7 cm in length and 5 cm in height. It is narrow transversely, measuring approximately 1.5 cm at the floor and 1–2 mm at the roof.

## VESTIBULE

It is the entrance of the nasal cavity from the nostrils and is lined by skin containing hair follicles. It forms part of the dangerous area of face because of the presence of the retrograde venous drainage through ophthalmic veins (without valves), which can lead to complications like cavernous sinus thrombosis. The vestibule is demarcated from the nasal mucosa by the limen nasi, which corresponds to the superior margin of the lower lateral cartilage.

## COLUMELLA

It is the part between the two nasal vestibules and forms the caudal end of the nasal septum. It is formed by the medial crurae of the two lower lateral cartilages. The lower lateral cartilages and the caudal end of the septum support the tip of the nose. Injury of any form to either caudal septum or lower lateral cartilages will change the shape of the tip.

## Framework of the Nasal Cavity

*In an articulated skull, the following bones/ cartilages bind each nasal cavity*

1. **The floor is formed by:**
   a. Palatine process of the maxilla.
   b. Horizontal process of the palatine bone.
2. **The roof consists of:**
   a. Cribriform plate of the ethmoid.
   b. Nasal process of the frontal bone.
   c. Body of the sphenoid.
3. **The medial wall is formed by:**
   a. Cartilaginous nasal septum
   b. Bony nasal septum
   c. Membranous columella.
4. **Lateral wall consists of:**
   a. Medial wall of the maxilla
   b. Inferior concha
   c. Middle and superior concha of the ethmoid bone.

## MEDIAL WALL (NASAL SEPTUM)

This is formed by bony and cartilaginous framework and is lined by the mucoperiosteum and the mucoperichondrium respectively. This forms the bulk of the nasal septum. The small caudal part is membranous (columella) and is lined by skin.

Following structures form the bony nasal septum (Figs 1.3 and 1.4).

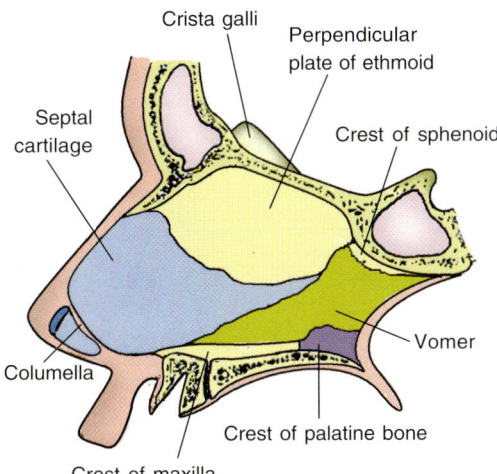

**Fig. 1.3:** Bony and cartilaginous part of the nasal septum

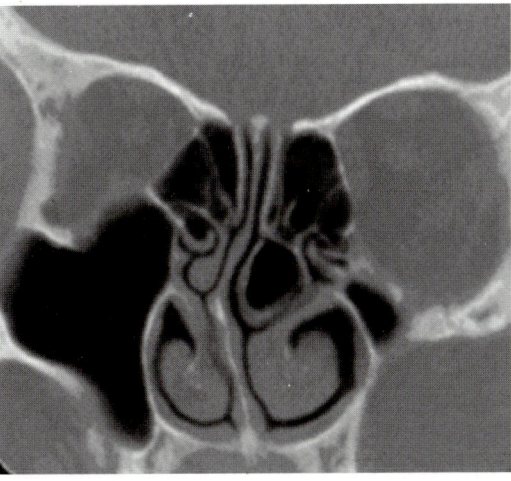

**Fig. 1.4a:** CT scan of the nose and paranasal sinus

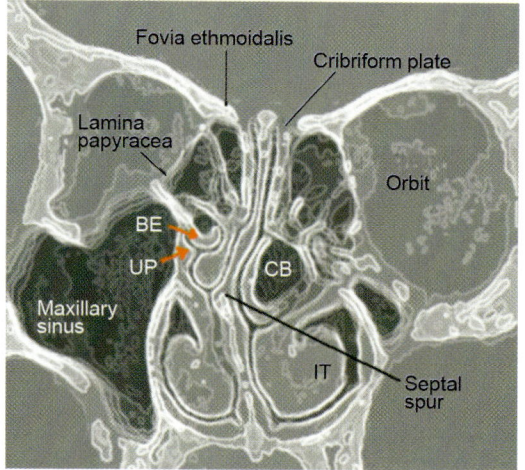

**Fig. 1.4b:** Same CT restructured showing the details

*Major contribution from*
- Perpendicular plate of ethmoid
- Vomer
- Palatine crest
- Maxillary crest

*Small contribution from*
- Nasal spine of the frontal bone
- Rostrum of the sphenoid
- Anterior nasal spine of the maxilla

The **cartilaginous** part of the nasal septum is formed by quadrangular cartilage with a contribution from upper and lower lateral cartilages.

**Membranous columella:** It is the membranous part of the septum between the medial crus of the lower lateral cartilage and the quadrangular cartilage. It is lined by skin and the floor does not have much relevance with respect to endoscopic sinus surgery, except that a deviated septum is associated with corresponding changes in the size and shape of the turbinate on the lateral wall.

The roof of nasal cavity is curved with concave surface downwards and is 7–8 cm long. The middle part is formed by the cribriform plate of ethmoid and is nearly horizontal. The anterior and posterior parts are sloping. The anterior part is formed by the nasal part of frontal bone, the nasal bone and by the junction of the lateral and septal cartilages.

The posterior part consists of the anterior and inferior surfaces of the body of the sphenoid and the bones in contact with these surfaces.

## Lateral Wall of the Nasal Cavity

Compared to the simple medial wall, the lateral wall is complicated in its anatomy. It bounds most of the paranasal sinuses and receives the openings from these sinuses (Figs 1.4 and 1.5).

The external nares lead to the skin lined part of the lateral nasal wall, the vestibule. This corresponds to the ala of the nose and is separated from the rest of the lateral wall (lateral wall proper) by a ridge, limen nasi or limen vestibuli which is formed by the lower end of upper lateral cartilage.

The lateral wall proper, lined by mucosa, bears 3 or 4 nasal conchae or turbinates, which are delicate projecting scrolls of bone covered by mucous membrane (Fig. 1.5).

These are named from below to upwards—inferior, middle and superior conchae. The fourth one, the supreme concha, is present unilaterally or bilaterally in 60% of cases. This is the smallest of all and is usually a mere ridge. The air spaces beneath and lateral to the conchae are termed meati which are named according to turbinates to which they are related, viz. inferior, middle and superior meati. The supreme meatus when present is usually a barely perceptible furrow below supreme concha. The part of the nasal cavity above the uppermost concha and below the body of sphenoid bone is the sphenoethmoidal recess.

All the anterior group of sinuses, viz. the frontal, anterior and middle ethmoid and maxillary sinuses drain into the middle meatus. The posterior group of sinuses, i.e. the posterior ethmoid and sphenoid drain above the middle turbinate. The sphenoid sinus drains into the sphenoethmoidal recess and the posterior ethmoids into the superior or supreme meatus (Figs 1.5 and 1.6).

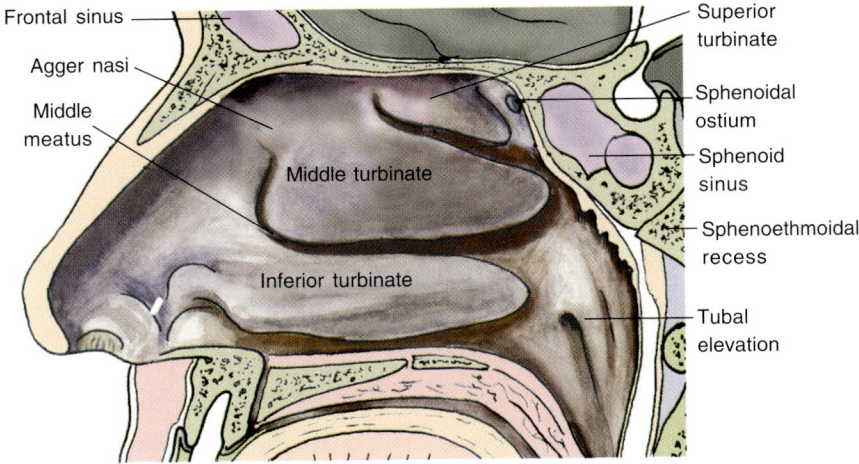

**Fig. 1.5:** Anatomy of the lateral nasal wall

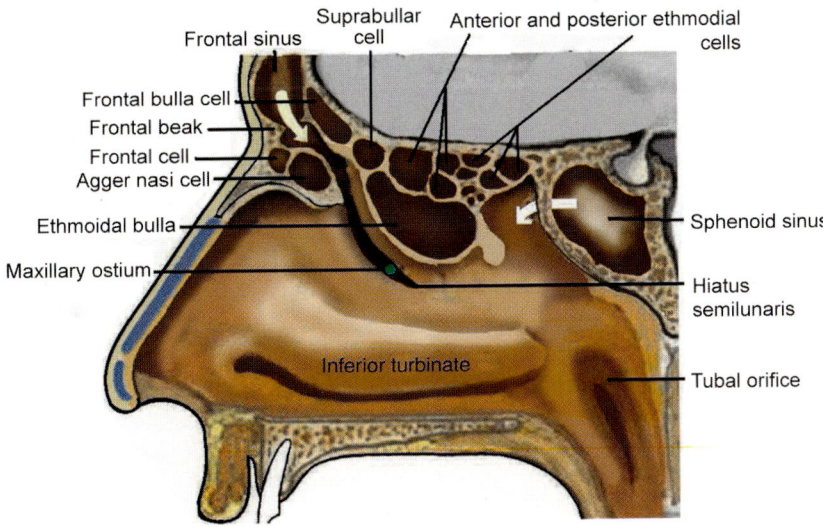

**Fig. 1.6:** Endoscopic anatomy of the lateral nasal wall and middle meatus

Both inferior and middle conchae begin anteriorly approximately at the level of the vertical plane of the forehead and extend one below the other almost to the choana.

Anterior to these two conchae, the lateral wall of nose above the limen nasi is more delicately marked, i.e.

1. About halfway between the anterior end of the middle concha and the dorsum of the nose is a slight projection, the agger nasi. It is said to be the remnant of additional concha found in lower animals, but is more important in man as it marks the location of anterior most of the anterior ethmoid cells called agger nasi cells.

2. The passageway above the agger nasi, the olfactory sulcus, leads to the olfactory area (dangerous area of nose).

3. Below and posterior to the agger nasi, it leads to the middle meatus proper through a shallow depression known as atrium of the middle meatus. This is situated above and anterior to the attached end of inferior turbinate.

The superior concha, about half the length of the other two, begins at about the middle of these. The 3 conchae converge somewhat towards each other posteriorly and the remaining part of the nasal cavity behind their posterior ends is the nasopharyngeal meatus. This opens into the nasopharynx through the choana. Sphenopalatine foramen is situated in the nasopharyngeal meatus, just midway between posterior ends of middle and superior turbinates. The vessels and nerves here can be traced towards the foramen and their vanishing point helps to locate the foramen.

## Inferior Nasal Concha and Inferior Meatus

Inferior nasal concha is an independent bone covered with thick mucous membrane which contains a vascular, cavernous plexus.

It is so arched that the inferior meatus is narrow anteriorly and posteriorly, but is both wider and higher at the junction of anterior and middle one-third of inferior turbinate. Here the attachment of inferior turbinate curves sharply, called the genu of inferior turbinate.

The nasolacrimal duct opens into the inferior meatus, in its most cephalic part, under the genu of inferior turbinate and is about 15–20 mm from limen nasi and 30–40 mm from the anterior nares. Nasolacrimal duct dysfunction rarely results from surgery of inferior meatus, just under the genu.

The nasolacrimal duct rarely opens lower in the inferior meatus and in such cases the orifice is slit-like, as the duct runs obliquely through the mucous membrane. Here it is usually protected by a fold of mucous membrane, the plica lacrimalis or the valve of Hasner.

## Middle Nasal Concha and Middle Meatus

The lateral wall of nasal cavity above the inferior turbinate is basically formed by the ethmoid labyrinth. Middle nasal concha is a part of the ethmoid labyrinth.

The attachment of middle turbinate to the lateral wall has 2 slopes, the ascending and the descending rami which meet at an angle, the genu of middle turbinate. The genu is situated anteriorly. The highest part of the middle meatus lies below the genu and is known as the frontal recess (Holinshead).

The insertion of the middle turbinate into the lateral wall is called axilla. Creating a flap in this region (axillary flap) can overcome the problem in accessing the frontal recess and the frontal sinus (Wormald, 2002).

The prominent structures in the middle meatus from the anterior to posterior are the uncinate process, the hiatus semi-lunaris and the bulla ethmoidalis.

The uncinate process is a crescent shaped ledge of bone, part of the ethmoid, and its posterior free and sharp margin form the anterior margin of a semilunar opening, the hiatus semilunaris. The bulla ethmoidalis, a rounded projection of the middle meatus, contains one or more ethmoid cells with their delicate walls. These cells are known variously as middle ethmoid or bullar cells. Some consider it as a part of anterior ethmoid.

The recess above the bulla is called suprabullar recess. Part of middle meatus posterosuperior to bulla and anterior to the posterior part of middle turbinate is called sinus lateralis.

The hiatus semilunaris leads to a groove between the uncinate process and bulla and is called ethmoidal infundibulum or uncinate or unciform groove. The ethmoidal infundibulum from the hiatus semilunaris extends downwards and forwards and varies in depth from 0.5 to 10 mm (average 5 mm) and therefore the upwardly projecting uncinate process varies in its height. Removal of uncinate process during endoscopic sinus surgery (ESS) exposes the infundibulum (Infundibulotomy).

*Boundaries of ethmoidal infundibulum:* It is a three-dimensional space and is bounded as follows:

*Anteriorly and superiorly:* Frontal process of maxilla.

*Anteromedial and anteroinferiorly:* Uncinate process, and the mucosa lining over it.

*Posteriorly:* Bulla ethmoidalis.

*Medially:* Communicates with middle meatus through the hiatus semilunaris, which forms the super medial boundary.

*Laterally:* Lamina papyracea and the lacrimal bone superiorly and the maxillary fontanellae inferiorly.

The relationship of infundibulum to frontal recess is determined by the attachment of the uncinate process. Based on the attachment superiorly with different situations, the uncinate process can be divided as: Type-A if inserts at the lamina papyracea, Type-B if inserts at the skull base and Type-C if inserts at the middle turbinate (Fig. 1.7a). The postero-inferior one third of the infundibulum receives the natural ostium of the maxillary sinus which is formed by part of the maxillary fontanellae (Fig. 1.7b).

The term frontal recess was first used by Killian in 1898. A true frontonasl duct does not exist. Mosher described connection between frontal sinus and anterior ethmoid as a recess. The frontal recess is bounded laterally by the lamina papyracea, medially by the middle turbinate, anteriorly the agger nasi cell and posteriorly the ethmoidal bulla cells. Van Alyea found the relationship of anterior ethmoidal cells to frontal recess besides agger nasi and termed these cells frontal cells. Agger nasi cell can vary in size and thus can affect the drainage pathway within the frontal recess. Kuhn (1996) classified frontal cells into four different types, the modification of this includes (Fig. 1.7c):

**Type-1:** Single cell above the agger nasi,
**Type-2:** Tier of cells above the agger nasi,
**Type-3:** Cells extending cephalad into the frontal sinus through the ostium but not extending 50% beyond the vertical height.
**Type-4:** Frontal cell that extends more than 50% beyond the vertical height.
**Frontal bulla cell:** Cell that extends from the suprabullar recess into the frontal sinus along the posterior wall.

Because of the variation in the development of the agger nasi and the frontal cell, the frontal recess surgery is quite challenging and the surgeon needs to have the thorough knowledge and prior radiological evaluation should be done before carefully uncapping these cells to clear the disease from the frontal recess and the frontal sinus.

The medial wall of maxillary sinus is partially membranous in the posterior part of middle meatus and is called the maxillary hiatus. This is divided into anterior and posterior fontanellae by the ethmoidal process of the inferior turbinate (Fig. 1.7b). The maxillary sinus opens at the junction of anterior and posterior fontanellae. At the fontanellae, the maxillary sinus mucosa and nasal mucosa are coated with no intervening bone. Any dehiscence in the fontanellae presents as an accessory ostium, thus creating an additional opening into the infundibulum.

Posteriorly and inferiorly the infundibulum becomes continuous with the middle meatus. Myerson demonstrated that the constant guide to cannulation of maxillary ostium is the angle formed by divergence of the uncinate process and bulla from one another in the posterior part of infundibulum.

The frontal sinus drains either directly into the infundibulum through nasofrontal duct or indirectly into the infundibulum through the anterior ethmoid cells.

The anterior ethmoid cells drain either into the infundibulum (at the frontoethmoidal recess) or anterior to it through the uncinate process (frontal recess of middle meatus).

The middle ethmoid cells open upon or above the bulla (suprabullar recess).

The opinion regarding the location and configuration of maxillary sinus ostium varies with different pioneers.

Myerson (1932) imagined a three-dimensional relationship of maxillary ostium. He opined that the internal ostium leads into a tubular *intranasal channel* of varying configuration depending on the development of uncinate process and bulla. He recognized that the ostium is located immediately below the orbital floor and the lamina papyracea, and perforating the lateral wall of infundibulum superior to ostium violates the orbit.

Van Alyea (1936) found maxillary ostium situated posteriorly in the infundibulum in two-thirds of cases, in the middle in one-

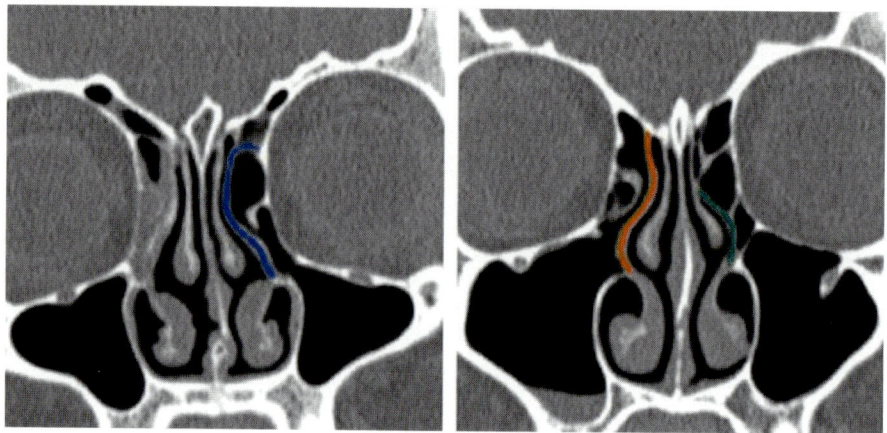

CT scans showing various types of uncinate process: Type-A (•), Type-B (•), Type-C (•)

**Fig. 1.7a:** Different types of uncinate process

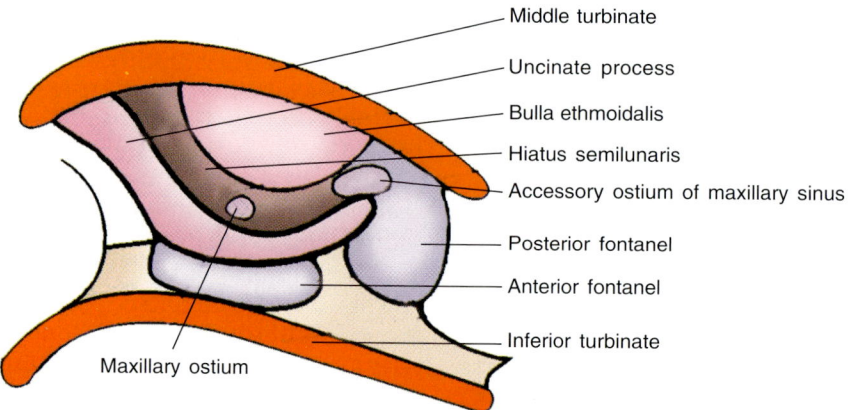

- Middle turbinate
- Uncinate process
- Bulla ethmoidalis
- Hiatus semilunaris
- Accessory ostium of maxillary sinus
- Posterior fontanel
- Anterior fontanel
- Inferior turbinate
- Maxillary ostium

**Fig. 1.7b:** Anatomy of the middle meatus

fourth of cases and in the anterior in 70% of cases. He found that the ostium was easily accessible for cannulation in only 40% of specimens.

When viewed from inside the antrum, the internal ostium is situated just 2–3 mm below the junction of medial wall and roof of the sinus, roughly half distance between anterior and posterior walls and about 4 cm from the floor of the antrum. When peered through the ostium towards the nasal cavity, uncinate process is seen anterosuperiorly and bulla posterosuperiorly.

The accessory sinus ostium when present is usually situated posterior to the natural ostium, even though endoscopically due to

illusory effect, it appears inferior to natural ostium. Van Alyea found accessory ostium in 23%, Myerson in 31%, Schaeffer in 43%, and Neivert in 25% of specimens.

Thus from the functional standpoint, the infundibular space represents the confluence of drainage from frontal, anterior and middle ethmoidal and maxillary sinuses. The infundibulum like the stem of a funnel collects the drainage from the anterior group of sinuses and opens into the middle meatus through the hiatus semilunaris. All these micro channels are situated in the anterior and middle ethmoid sinuses and hence any anatomical and pathological variation here causes diseases in dependent sinuses (Fig. 1.8).

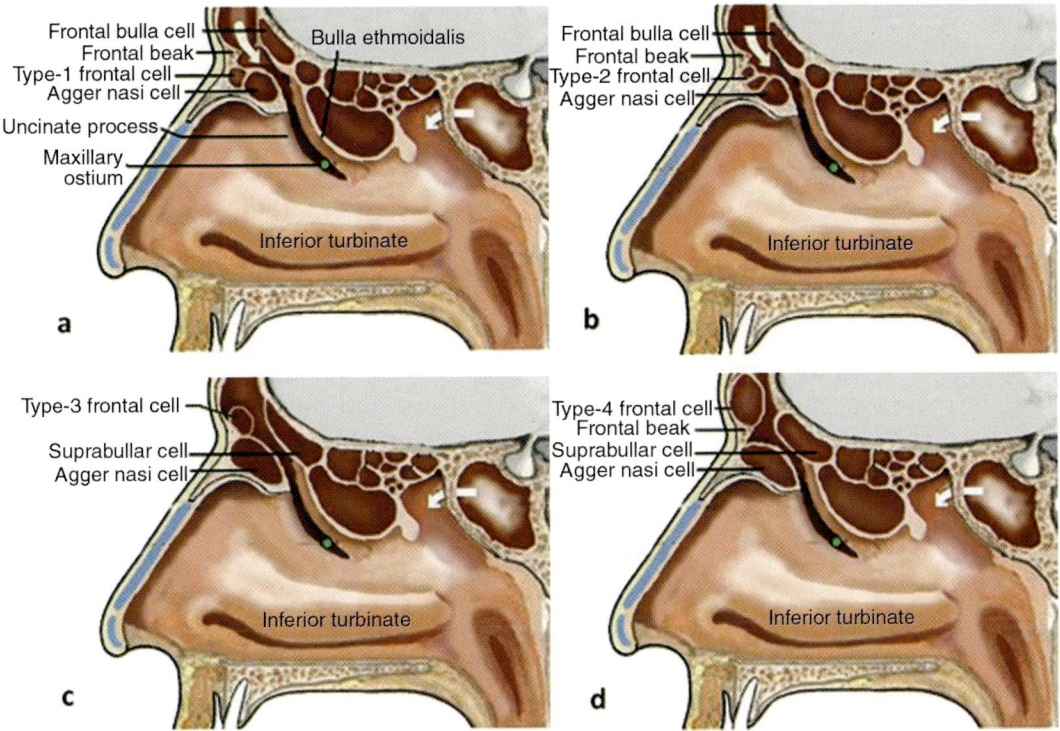

**Fig. 1.7c:** Four types of frontal cells: (a) Type-1, (b) Type 2, (c) Type 3, (d) Type 4, classified by Kuhn in1996

Noting this clinical significance, Naumann in 1965 described the anterior ethmoid-middle meatus complex as **osteomeatal unit** (Fig. 1.8).

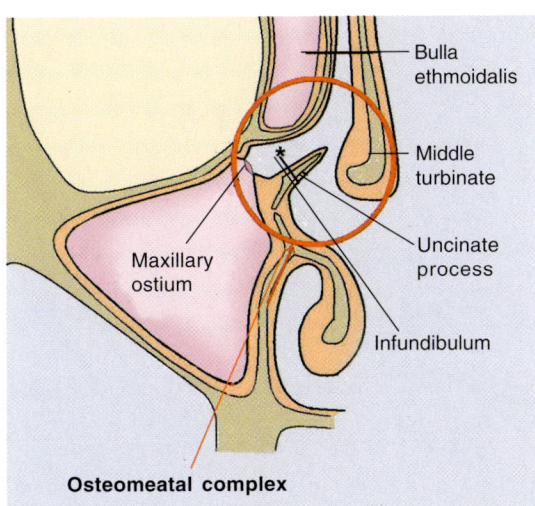

**Fig. 1.8:** The cross-sectional anatomy of osteomeatal complex

## Osteology of Lateral Nasal Wall

### Mainly formed by 2 bones

1. Ethmoid labyrinth
2. Inferior nasal concha

### Other bones participating

1. Medial wall of maxillary antrum
2. The lacrimal bone
3. Nasal bone
4. Frontal process of maxilla
5. Palatine bone (vertical lamina)

### PARANASAL SINUSES

They are air-filled spaces in the skull bones and are lined by mucosa, which drains into the nasal cavity by the mucociliary drainage. They are 8 in number, 4 on each side, namely the frontal, ethmoidal, maxillary and sphenoidal sinuses. The 4 pairs of paranasal sinuses are lined with ciliated, pseudo-stratified columnar epithelium. Goblet cells are inter-

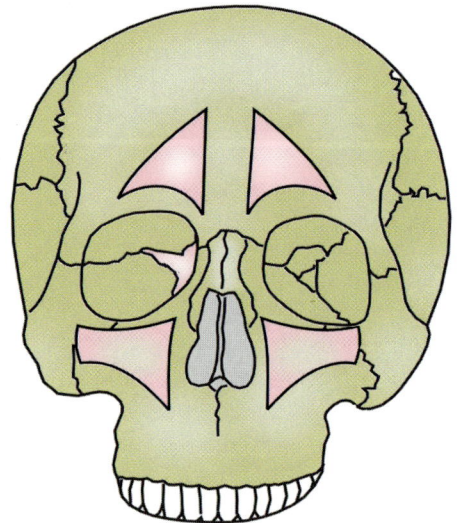

**Fig. 1.9:** Position of the anterior group of sinuses in the skull

spersed among the columnar cells. The mucosa is attached directly to the bone. Involvement

of the surrounding bone and further extension of the infection into the orbital and intracranial compartments occur in inadequately treated patients and in specific types of sinusitis such as fungal sinusitis (Fig. 1.9).

Functionally there are two groups
1. **Anterior group:** These drain into the middle meatus.
   a. Frontal sinus
   b. Maxillary sinus
   c. Anterior ethmoidal sinus
2. **Posterior group:** These drain into the superior meatus/sphenoethmoidal recess.
   a. Posterior ethmoidal sinus
   b. Sphenoid sinus.

## MAXILLARY SINUS (ANTRUM OF HIGHMORE)

This is a 3 sided pyramidal in shape. In an adult its capacity is approximately 15 ml (Fig. 1.10).

**Base (medial wall)** corresponds to the lateral wall of nasal cavity in relation to the middle

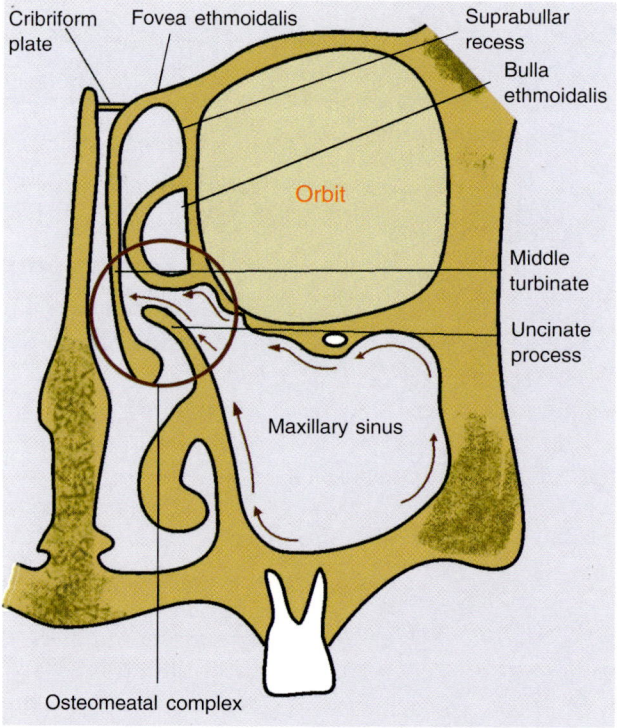

**Fig. 1.10:** Relations of maxillary sinus with respect to orbit, ethmoids and osteomeatal complex

and inferior turbinates. The ostium of the maxillary sinus opens in the medial wall into the middle meatus between the uncinate process and the bulla ethmoidalis as described under lateral wall of the nasal cavity.

Apex is directed towards zygomatic process.

**The three walls of this pyramid**

a. **Anterolateral wall** covered by the periosteum, soft tissue and skin of the cheek. It is relatively thinner in the canine fossa and is present lateral to the canine eminence. This site is used for approaching the maxillary sinus in Caldwell-Luc operation. This wall has an opening called infraorbital foramen, which is situated about one cm. below the infraorbital margin. Infraorbital nerve and vessels emerge through this foramen.

b. **Superior wall (roof of antrum)** is formed by orbital plate. This is covered by the orbital periosteum. At its midpoint in its inferior aspect is a groove, through which the infraorbital nerve and vessels pass before emerging out of the infraorbital foramen.

c. **Posterior wall** is formed by a thin plate of bone and is related to pterygopalatine fossa, which consists of third part of internal maxillary artery, vidian nerve and the sphenopalatine ganglion. Posteromedially the bone is attached to pterygoid plates with a dehiscence called the sphenopalatine foramen. This opens into the lateral wall of the nose just behind the posterior end of the middle turbinate. This transmits the sphenopalatine vessels and the nerves.

Floor is formed by alveolar and palatine process of the maxilla. It lies at or above the floor of the nasal cavity in a child while it lies at a lower level in an adult.

## FRONTAL SINUS

It is pyramidal in shape and its volume, size and shape is variable and can often be rudimentary. The 2 frontal sinuses are often asymmetrical in shape. Bony septa may partially sub-divide it into one or more compartments. Its average capacity is about 7 ml in adults. It is not present at birth and it usually develops after the age of about 5 years as an extension of the anterior ethmoidal air cell.

Development of this sinus varies markedly. It develops as one of the several outgrowths from the region of the frontal recess similar to the anterior ethmoidal cells. In fact some regard it as an anterior ethmoid cell that has invaded the frontal bone.

Several sinuses may occur on one or both sides, lying one lateral to other or one behind the other. These sinuses may either drain one into the other or drain separately.

Frontal bulla are cells that pneumatize from the anterior ethmoid into the frontal sinus. Two features distinguish a frontal bulla from a Kuhn type-3 cell:

• It is pneumatized from the region above the ethmoid bulla and along the skull base into the frontal sinus.

• Its posterior wall is formed by the skull base. Its anterior wall directly faces the interior of the frontal sinus.

Frontal bullae may narrow the frontal recess from the posterior side. When combined with agger nasi and Kuhn cells, they may contribute to the obstruction of ventilation and drainage (Leunig, 2008).

Important relations of frontal sinus are the anterior cranial fossa and the orbit. The bone separating the sinus from the above is usually thin and thus an operative perforation can easily occur.

## Frontonasal Connections

The drainage of frontal sinus is highly variable and depends on its development, i.e. whether it originates in frontal recess directly or from one or more anterior ethmoid cells arising in frontal pits.

According to Kasper's investigations, the frontal sinus drained into the frontoethmoidal recess directly in 4% of cases and indirectly through the infundibular anterior ethmoidal cells in 34% of cases. In 62% it drained via the anterior ethmoidal cell into the area below the genu of middle turbinate either anterior,

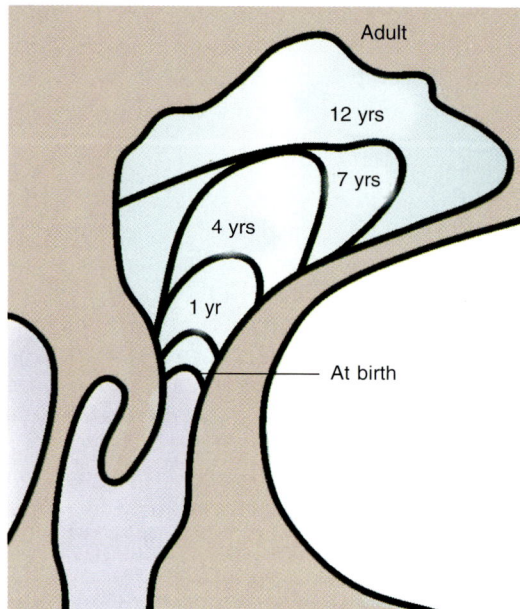

Fig. 1.11: Size and extent of the frontal sinus at various age

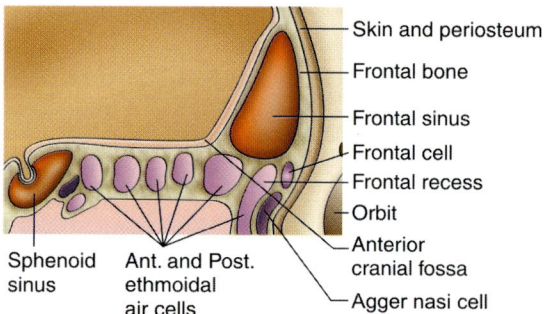

Fig. 1.12: Relation of the frontal sinus

posterior or superior to the frontoethmoidal recess.

Van Alyea opined that anatomical variations such as frontal bulla and blocked middle meatus caused by impingement of middle turbinate head against lateral wall were the commonest causes of chronic frontal sinusitis (Fig. 1.11).

### Position

It is situated between the inner and outer table of the frontal bone. It occupies variable amount of frontal bone.

Floor is formed by orbital roof. As it is relatively thin, it is used as a surgical approach.

Medially it is separated from the other frontal sinus by a thin interfrontal septum.

Posterior wall is related to anterior cranial fossa.

Anterior wall is covered by periosteum and skin of the forehead (Fig. 1.12).

### ETHMOIDAL SINUSES

It is well developed in children and it occupies the medial wall of the orbit and upper third of the lateral wall of the nose. It consists of 7 to 15 cells on each side and is divided into 2 groups based on their drainage. The ethmoidal air cells are small and do not have regular disposition, symmetry or fixed number.

These are situated within the ethmoid labyrinth and separates the nasal cavity from orbit. The ethmoid labyrinth is roughly pyramid shaped with the base posteriorly in relation to sphenoid and apex anteriorly limited by the frontal process of maxilla and nasal process of frontal bone.

It is about 4–5 cm long (anteroposterior), 2.5–3 cm high and about 0.5 cm wide anteriorly and 1.5 cm posteriorly. Thus as a whole, the ethmoid labyrinth forms a thin plate broader posteriorly and thinner anteriorly.

Superiorly, the labyrinthine roof is thicker and is called fovea ethmoidalis. This is limited anteriorly by the inferior wall of frontal sinus and posteriorly by the sphenoidal bone. Superior wall of ethmoid labyrinth/the ethmoidal roof is formed by fovea ethmoidalis and is related to the anterior cranial fossa. The fovea slopes medially and downward. Its medial part is thinner and may be easily injured. The fovea is at a higher level than the cribriform plate, especially in its lateral part.

Laterally it is related to the orbit and the lacrimal sac and is separated by a papery thin bone called lamina papyracea.

Posterolaterally it is related to the sphenoid sinus. The posterior ethmoid cells may extend lateral to the sphenoid sinus where it is related to the optic nerve. These cells are called the *Onodi cells.*

Medially the ethmoid labyrinth is related to nasal cavity.

The lateral wall of the ethmoidal labyrinth are attached to several bones that are related to the optic nerve, orbit and the lacrimal sac. They are extremely important to the surgeon as they can be injured or can be surgically approached through this wall. They include frontal bone lying anteriorly and above, lacrimal bone (OS unguis) anteriorly and below. Immediately posterior to these two structures is the lamina papyracea (OS planum) above that separates the orbit and the medial wall of maxilla and the vertical lamina of the palatine bone below.

Inferiorly ethmoid has no wall. Its lower limits are marked by the opening of middle meatus and can therefore be considered the horizontal plane passing along the lower margin of middle turbinate.

The medial wall of ethmoid labyrinth consists above of a continuous lamina called turbinate lamina and below of ridges called turbinates (middle, superior and supreme) and corresponding meat.

The medial wall has 5 principal lamellae which penetrate into the labyrinth towards the lateral wall. They are 1. uncinate process, 2. bulla, 3. middle turbinate, 4. superior turbinate and 5. supreme turbinate (Fig. 1.13).

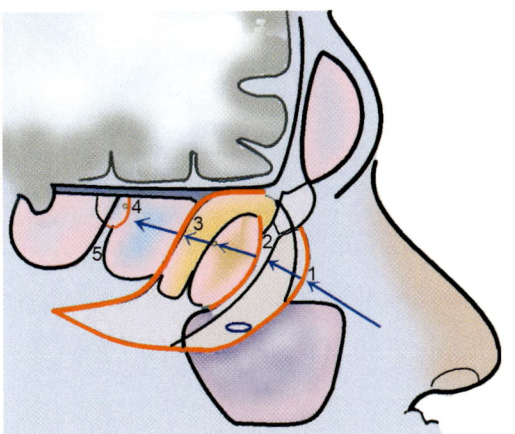

**Fig. 1.13:** Five principal lamellae of the medial wall of ethmoid

The more delicate secondary lamellae are placed irregularly between the primary ones, giving rise to multiple ethmoid cells.

1. **Uncinate process lamella** is crescent shaped, curves downwards and backwards with the concave free sharp margin facing upwards. It is inserted obliquely into the external wall forming part of the infundibular canal. The lower free edge is secured from front to back to the frontal process of maxilla, lacrimal bone and maxillary sinus medial wall immediately above the attachment of inferior turbinate.

   The uncinate process lamella posteriorly terminates in a partially membranous wall of maxilla (fontanellae) where it splits onto several slender extensions which reinforce the membranous wall.

2. **Bullar lamella:** Few millimeters behind and above the uncinate process is a second arched lamella which forms a dome-shaped protuberance called the bulla ethmoidalis. This lamella is applied laterally on the papyraceous lamina. Posteriorly it is attached to the front of the middle turbinate lamella, forming a sulcus, the suprabullar sulcus.

3. **The middle turbinate lamella** is the least variable. It consists of 2 parts: one lateral (lamina basilaris) and another medial (lamina recurvata), perpendicular to each other. The lamina basilaris (ground lamella) forming the posterior part of middle turbinate runs obliquely downwards and backwards from the anterior ethmoid roof to a small crest of palatine bone (vertical branch) near sphenopalatine foramen, towards the lateral surface of the labyrinth (lamina papyracea). The lamina basilaris separates the middle and posterior ethmoidal cells.

   The lamina recurvata forming the anterior part of middle turbinate ascends upwards lining medially the ethmoid air cells and is attached to the roof of ethmoid at the junction of fovea with cribriform plate.

   The lamina recurvata thus forms the anterior part of the turbinate lamina. The middle turbinate thus has 2 attachments:

- To the lamina papyracea via basal lamina.
- To the ethmoid roof (junction of fovea and cribriform plate) via lamina recurvata.

4. **The superior turbinate lamella** (present in 85% of cases). This divides the posterior ethmoidal cells into 2 groups, one above and one below the lamella.

5. **Lamella of the sphenoid sinus:** The ethmoids during their development have tendency to grow steadily in all directions beyond the confines of ethmoid until deterred by hard compact bone. The cells which reside within the ethmoid bone are termed intramural cells and those outside are called extramural cells. Thus the ethmoid cells may invade the supraorbital plate of frontal bone, infraorbital plate of maxilla, the middle turbinate (concha bullosa), the sphenoid and lacrimal bone. The frontal sinus is considered by some as part of ethmoid which has invaded the frontal sinus.

The extent of pneumatization has definite implication in an endoscopic sinus surgery.

The anterior group of cells, according to Bagatella *et al.* consists of 2–10 cells, their number being inversely proportional to their size. They are topographically divided into 4 subgroups from front to back as:

1. **Preinfundibular cell** (0–1)

2. **Lateral infundibular cells** (0–2) situated lateral to infundibulum, between the frontal process of maxilla, floor of frontal sinus and lacrimal bone. In over pneumatized state, these can invade the above bones.

3. **Postinfundibular cells** (0–2) situated posterior to infundibulum and anterior to bulla, between the papyraceous lamina and the floor of frontal sinus.

4. **The bullar cells** (2–5)

The posterior ethmoidal cells are of two types:

1. Intramural cells, which are located within the ethmoid bone.

2. Extramural cells, which are located in the adjacent bones like maxilla and sphenoid bones, like Haller cells, Onodi cells.

The posterior ethmoidal cells are situated behind the level of the basal lamella and above the horizontal attachment of the middle turbinate to the lateral nasal wall. The posterior ethmoid cells are large and more rectangular in shape with their lateral wall in close contact with optic nerve. At a lower level, the sphenoid rostrum, protrudes into the posterior ethmoid cells at the midline like the nose cone of a rocket. Thus here the sphenoid ostium is surrounded by the posterior ethmoidal cells.

Here, the surgeon who tries to enter the sphenoid through the posterior ethmoid, has to be cautious not to mistake the junction the sphenoid rostrum and roof of posterior ethmoid cells for the anterior sphenoidal wall. If mistaken, a craniotomy could be performed.

## SPHENOIDAL SINUS

This is situated in the body of sphenoid. The sinuses of the two sides are divided by an asymmetrically placed median intersphenoidal septum. The sphenoid sinus drains into the sphenoethmoidal recess. It is related to a number of important structures because of its situation in the skull.

This sinus appears and begins to grow only after 3rd year and actually excavate the body of sphenoid. The degree of pneumatisation of this sinus is highly variable. Its capacity is said to vary from 0.5 to 30 ml (av 7.5 ml).

The sinus either may be limited to body of sphenoid, or it may extend to the other parts of sphenoid, namely the greater and lesser wings, anterior clinoid process, pterygoid process, etc. and also to the basilar portion of the occipital bone. As the degree of pneumatisation increases, the surrounding vital relations like optic nerve, ICA, maxillary nerve, etc. are brought more into the sinus cavity producing corresponding bulges into the cavity. ESS in such state is more dangerous.

The sphenoid sinus opens into the sphenoethmoidal recess (Fig. 1.6) usually through the posterior wall of the recess. Occasionally it may open through the lateral wall of the recess.

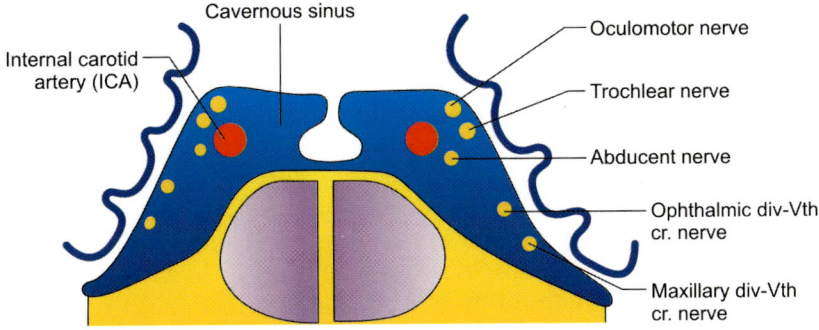

**Fig. 1.14:** Relations of the sphenoid sinus and contents of the cavernous sinus

## Relations (Fig. 1.14)

### Superiorly

1. Pituitary gland bulges into the sphenoid sinus posterosuperiorly. This is often used as a surgical approach (transsphenoidal hypophysectomy).
2. Optic chiasma
3. Olfactory tract
4. Frontal lobe of the brain

### Anteriorly

1. Sphenopalatine foramen
2. Sphenoidal crest
3. Nasal cavity

### Inferiorly

1. Nasopharynx and choana
2. Vidian nerve is situated inferolaterally and its position helps in vidian neurectomy.

### Posteriorly

1. Basilar artery
2. Brainstem

### Laterally

1. Cavernous sinus and its contents (III, IV, V and VI cranial nerves).
2. Internal carotid artery

## Vital Relations of Sphenoethmoidal Sinuses

### Orbit

The ethmoid labyrinth is separated from the orbit by only a thin bone 'the lamina papyracea'. Apart from this, the lamina may have natural dehiscences especially in the two cranial quarters. This permits infection to spread from ethmoids to orbit (5.6% in Kozlov's series and 14/1188 skulls in Zuckerlandl's series had natural dehiscences).

The inferomedial aspect of lamina papyracea forms the lateral boundary of ethmoid infundibulum in close relation to the maxillary sinus ostium.

Thus an attempt to perform middle meatal antrostomy superior to the natural ostium violates the orbit.

A previous ethmoid surgery is likely to have distorted the nasal anatomy, and also could have caused dehiscence in the lamina, thus making prone to orbital injury during ESS (Fig. 1.15).

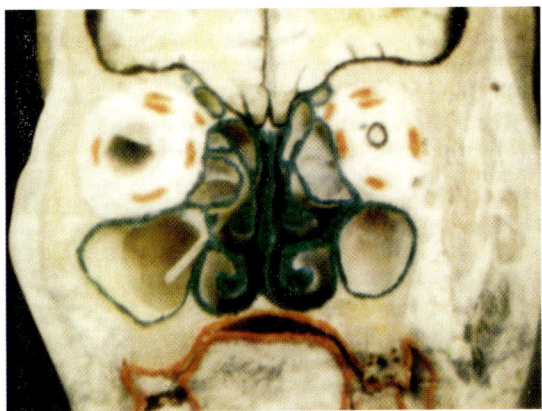

**Fig. 1.15:** Relations of ethmoid and orbit shown in a cadaveric specimen (coronal section)

Injury to the lamina at the plane of anterior ethmoid artery could cause injury to medial and superior rectus causing diplopia.

## Optic Nerve

This lies in close apposition to the lateral aspect of posterior ethmoid and sphenoid. The optic canal varying in length from 5.5 to 11.5 mm (av 9.22 mm) runs between the two roots of the lesser wing of sphenoid after coming in relation to posterior ethmoid.

Its distal opening termed the optic ring borders on the most posterior ethmoid cells in about 50% of cases, on the sphenoid sinus in 25% and on the partition separating the two sinuses in other 25% of cases. Thus, in nearly 75% of cases, the optic nerve is not only in close relationship with sphenoid sinus, but also with the ethmoid sinus as well. In 25% of cases, the nerve is almost completely surrounded by an air space (Fig. 1.16).

During its course, the optic nerve produces against the superolateral wall of sphenoid, a bulge called optic bulge which is more pronounced in over pneumatised sphenoid cells. Such eminence was missing in only one of the 50% specimens investigated by Fuji *et al*. They found that 78% of specimens had less than a 0.5 mm thickness of bone separating the nerve from sinus and dehiscence were present in 4%. Similar findings were observed by Maniscalco and Habal (1978), Meloni *et al*.

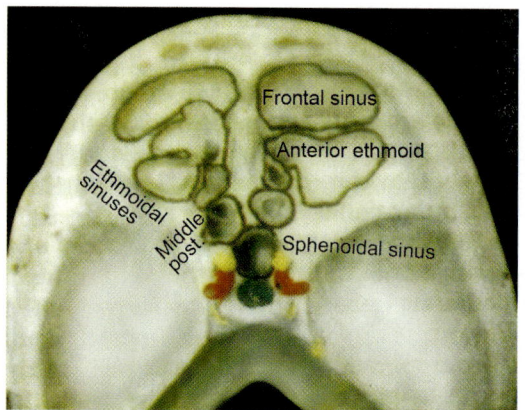

**Fig. 1.16:** Vital relations of sphenoid and ethmoids shown in cadaveric specimen (axial sections)

observed optic eminence with extremely thin bone in 70% patients by axial CT scans.

## Internal Carotid Artery

Similar to optic nerve, the internal carotid artery can also produce bulges into the sphenoid sinus.

Van Alyea found 65% of arteries bulging into the sinus. In 14% the whole serpentine course of vessel could be tracked along the lateral sinus wall. Renn and Rhoton (1975) reported carotid prominence in 71% of specimens. In 66% the thickness of bone separating the artery from sinus was less than 1 mm and dehiscence were noticed in 4%. According to Fuji *et al*. the bony layer separating was thinner than 0.5 mm in 88% of specimens and dehiscence found in 8%. Teatani *et al*. observed carotid prominence in 72% of axial CT scans.

## Lacrimal Sac and Nasolacrimal Duct

The medial wall of lacrimal sac roughly corresponds to the atrium of the middle meatus. The anterior ethmoid cells may invade the lacrimal bone and in such conditions the lacrimal sac is vulnerable to injury by an ESS which is very rare.

The nasolacrimal duct runs from the lacrimal fossa downwards but slightly backwards and laterally and lies in a bony wall (nasolacrimal canal) between the maxillary sinus and nasal cavity. In the canal the duct is closely fused to the periosteum.

Whitnall found close contact between anterior ethmoidal cells and upper half of lacrimal fossa in all 100 orbits he examined, and in more than half of these the fossa was directly related to these cells. The lower half of the fossa was found, in every instance, directly related to the middle meatus.

The nasolacrimal duct may be injured during a middle meatal antrostomy when the ostium is enlarged anteriorly with a backbiting forceps. The duct lies 8–17 mm (av 10 mm) anterior to the ostium and approximately 5 mm from the anterior border of the membranous anterior fontanellae.

## Anterior Ethmoidal Artery

The anterior and posterior ethmoidal arteries leave the orbit through their respective foramina in the frontoethmoid suture line, approximately 24 and 36 mm respectively from anterior lacrimal crest. The arteries cross across the sinus having a brief intracranial course and enter the nose through their own foramina just below the cribriform plate.

During the intracranial course, at the skull base, the anterior ethmoidal artery runs in a partial or complete bony conduit at the junction of anterior and middle ethmoid cells, usually being attached to the ethmoidal roof by a bony septum.

This artery is a useful landmark during FESS as it indicates the level of fovea and thus the superior limit of ethmoidectomy. The artery is likely to be injured during ESS.

## Anterior Cranial Fossa

The cribriform plate and the fovea separate the anterior cranial fossa from nasal cavity and ethmoids respectively.

The cribriform plate is the most dependent portion of the anterior cranial fossa and forms the roof of the nasal cavity. It is perforated by nerve filaments of the olfactory nerve. Anteriorly the middle turbinate is attached to it by means of the planum recurvatum. This attachment is at the junction of fovea and cribriform plate.

The fovea ethmoidalis is the roof of the ethmoid labyrinth and lies at a higher level than cribriform plate. The former sharply dips down medially and gets attached to the latter. The medial aspect of fovea is very thin and can be easily damaged.

The surface of fovea is undulating and descends 15° from the horizontal as it passes posteriorly.

The level of cribriform plate is marked by the mid-pupillary line externally and by level of ethmoid foramina within the orbit.

The fovea ethmoidalis was found to be 4–7 mm higher than the level of cribriform plate in about 70%. Based on this depth, Keros (1962) described the olfactory fossa into three

types: Type-I (0–3 mm), Type-II (4–7 mm), Type-III (8–16 mm). Also the 2 cribriform plates could be found at different levels. During ethmoidectomy, staying lateral to the middle turbinate will prevent violation of cribriform plate. Traction to the mid-turbinate during nasal procedures may injure the cribriform plate.

Bone defects in the fovea have been reported. Kozlov observed them in 8.5% of 70 cadaver dissections. The dura is closely applied to the roof of the ethmoid and hence CSF leak easily occurs by injury to fovea. During ethmoidectomy, identify the fovea as yellowish bone. Anterior ethmoidal artery also suggests the level of fovea. Staying below this level helps in prevention of injury to fovea. At the region of anterior ethmoidal artery, the fovea was found to be 10 times thinner than the neighboring roof (Stammberger).

## Blood Supply of the Paranasal Sinuses

Infraorbital and superior dental arteries derived from the internal maxillary artery supply maxillary sinus.

Branches of the anterior and posterior ethmoidal artery supply ethmoidal sinus and frontal sinus.

Sphenoid sinus is supplied by pharyngeal branch of the internal maxillary artery.

## Development of the Nose and Paranasal Sinuses

Nose develops from a number of mesenchymal processes surrounding the primitive stomodeum. The frontonasal process arises between the central aspect of the forebrain and the epithelial roof of the mouth. A highly specialized ectodermal tissue called olfactory placode develops during the 5th week of intrauterine life, on each side of ventral surface of the frontonasal elevation. This divides it into median and lateral nasal processes. The olfactory placode sinks in to form the olfactory pit (Fig. 1.17).

The extension of the mesenchyme from the median process gives rise to premaxillary process of the developing mouth. This subsequently also forms the upper lip and

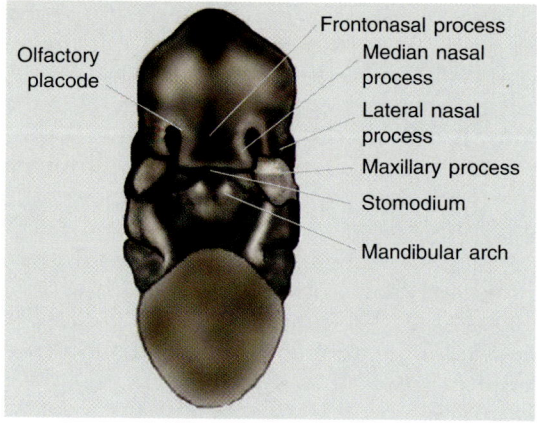

**Fig. 1.17:** Embryo showing early stage of nasal cavity and development of related structures

medial crus of the lower lateral cartilage. In the mean time another mesenchymal process, the maxillary process develops from the dorsal end of the mandibular arch and this fuses with the lateral nasal process, the two being separated by the naso-maxillary groove. Ectoderm along the boundaries of these two processes remains, giving rise to the nasolacrimal ridge from which the nasolacrimal duct arises later. The lateral nasal process forms the nasal bones, the upper lateral cartilages and the lateral crus of the lower lateral cartilages. The median maxillary process fuses with the median nasal elevation leading to the formation of the primitive external nares. From this a deepening pit in the mesenchyme produces the nasal cavity. The primitive nose and mouth are separated by the bucconasal membrane, which disappears later to facilitate communication posteriorly through a primitive choana. This is situated just behind the primitive palate. Failure to canalise leads to choanal atresia. Initially the external nares are widely separated but later come closer as the frontonasal process reduces gradually.

The primitive nasal septum is initially entirely cartilaginous. The superior portion undergoes ossification to form the perpendicular plate of the ethmoid. The premaxillary and the maxillary process establish the continuity with the primitive nasal septum, thus defining the two primitive nasal

cavities. On each side of the anterior nasal septum, an invagination of the ectoderm represents the vomeronasal organ. The vomer ossifies in the connective tissue covering the residual posterior inferior cartilage from two centers, which unite below the cartilage creating a deep grove in which the quadrilateral cartilage lodges. As the growth continues, the bony lamellae fuse and the cartilage gets absorbed. At puberty the lamellae are almost completely united with the everted alae. An anterior groove remains suggestive of the vomer's bi-lamellar origin. On the lateral wall of the nose a series of elevation appears within the nasal cavity at 6th week of intrauterine life, which ultimately forms the turbinates.

The primordial of the sinuses arises rather late during the prenatal period. The frontal sinus is the last to develop. In the first and second months of intrauterine life, the main features of the nasal cavities are defined. The paranasal sinuses arise as localized epithelial invaginations or recesses of the nasal mucosa, after the second month. These recesses become the ostia of the various sinuses. The maxillary sinus and sphenoidal sinus arise as mucosal recess during the 3rd prenatal month. The invagination developing from the hiatus semilunaris forms the future maxillary sinus. The ethmoidal cells originate during the 5th and 6th months of the IUL from the middle and superior meatus into anterior and posterior groups. They are divided into anterior and posterior groups respectively based on their origin. The frontal sinus (Fig. 1.11) develops after birth with lot of variation due to different source of origin like either direct extension of the frontal recess into the frontal bone, in which case the frontal sinus drainage pathway is through a distinct ostium (primary frontal sinus ostium) or if it is from the ethmoidal infundibulum and takes origin from one or more anterior ethmoidal cells, the drainage pathway is restricted to the frontonasal duct. The growth of surrounding ethmoidal cells can encroach upon the proximal part of the frontal sinus to compress the nasofrontal duct. The growth of surrounding ethmoidal cells can encroach the proximal part of the frontal sinus and can affect the development of frontal sinus and may even exceed the growth of primary frontal sinus and sometime can present as a bullous presentation called frontal bulla.

## ORBITAL ANATOMY

The orbit is closed related to the paranasal sinuses. The ethmoid sinus is separated from the orbit by a papery thin plate of bone called lamina papyracea. The lateral wall of the sphenoid sinus is closely related to the orbital apex and the optic nerve. Frontal sinus is related to the roof of the orbit and if over-pneumatized, the frontal sinus may even form the entire roof of the orbit. The roof of the maxillary sinus forms the floor of the orbit. Any inflammatory, traumatic or neoplastic lesion of the paranasal sinuses may complicate the orbit and similarly an orbital lesion may present in or could be surgically accessed through the sinuses. Moreover, the orbital anatomy is important for endoscopic sinus surgeon to perform endoscopic dacryocystorhinostomy.

Orbit is a quadrilateral pyramid with its base facing forwards, laterally and slightly inferiorly. The average volume of orbit is 30 ml, of which 70% is occupied by retrobulbar structures. Orbit is made up of seven bones, namely sphenoid, lacrimal, palatal, maxillary, ethmoid, frontal, and zygomatic. It has also seven important contents, namely the globe (7 ml), extraocular muscles (EOM), optic nerve, cranial nerves III, IV, V and VI, blood vessels, lacrimal gland and sac, orbital fat.

The orbit consists of 4 walls (Fig. 1.18)
- Medial
- Lateral
- Superior (roof)
- Inferior (floor)

## MEDIAL WALL

- It is composed of
  - Frontal process of maxilla
  - Lacrimal bone
  - Lamina papyracea of ethmoid
  - Body of sphenoid
- At the frontoethmoid suture, where the medial wall meets the roof, foramina for anterior and posterior ethmoidal vessels and nerves are located.
- Ethmoid foramina are also indicators of level of cribriform plate.
- Rule of 24-12-6 (Rontal *et al.*)
  - Distance from anterior lacrimal crest to anterior ethmoid foramen—24 mm
  - Distance from anterior to posterior ethmoid foramen—12 mm

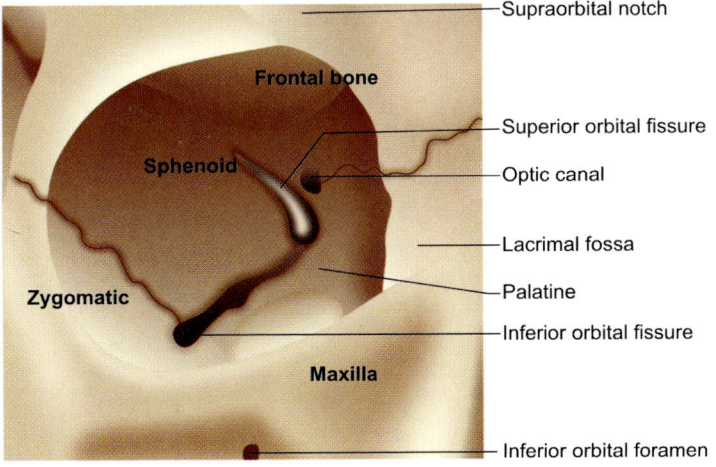

**Fig. 1.18:** Orbital anatomy

- Distance from posterior ethmoid foramen to optic canal—6 mm
- Lacrimal fossa for lacrimal sac lies between anterior and posterior lacrimal crests
- As the medial wall is thin in parts and could be dehiscent, there is risk for orbital cellulitis, from spread of paranasal sinus infection or mucocele.

## LATERAL WALL

- Greater wing of sphenoid
- Orbital surface of zygoma
- Zygomatic process of frontal bone
  - Posterior boundaries of lateral wall could be taken as the superior and inferior orbital fissures
  - Superior orbital fissure is about 28 mm from the fronto-zygomatic suture at the orbital rim
  - Optic nerve lies 8 mm behind the medial edge of the superior orbital fissure (SOF)
  - SOF extends posteriorly to the cavernous sinus
  - Lateral wall is encountered in
    - Orbital decompression
    - Lateral craniotomy
    - Infratemporal fossa surgery
    - Lateral orbitotomy
    - Exploration of fractures

## SUPERIOR WALL (ROOF)

- Triangular in shape and consists of:
  - Orbital plate of frontal bone
  - Lesser wing of sphenoid
- In the superomedial area of roof, 5 mm posterior to the orbital rim is the trochlea— a connective tissue sling anchoring the tendinous part of the superior oblique muscle to the orbit. Avoid injury to trochlea during surgery to prevent vertical diplopia.
- Supraorbital notch/foramen in the superior orbital margin transmitting supraorbital vessels and nerves.
- Superior walls is encountered in
  - Frontal sinus trephination

- External frontoethmoidectomy
- Orbital decompression
- Orbital fracture repair
- Orbital clearance/exenteration
- Faciocranial resection

## INFERIOR WALL (FLOOR)

- Composed of
  - Orbital plate of maxilla (Fig. 1.19)
  - Zygomatic orbital plate (anterolaterally)
- The infraorbital canal which transmits infraorbital nerve and artery is the thinnest and hence weakest part of the floor. It leads to the infraorbital foramen.
- Anteromedially just behind the orbital rim is a shallow depression for the origin of the inferior oblique muscle. Disruption of IO causes vertical diplopia.
- Floor is separated from lateral wall by inferior orbital fissure. It transmits infra-orbital nerve and artery, inferior ophthalmic vein and anterior/posterior superior alveolar nerves.
- It is encountered in
  - Orbital decompression
  - Repair of orbital floor fractures
  - Maxillectomy

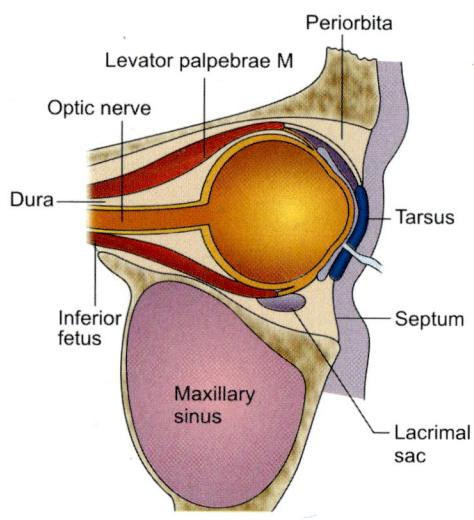

**Fig. 1.19:** Orbit and related structures

## PERIORBITA

- It is the periosteum lining the bony walls.
- It is continuous with the dura mater at the optic foramen and superior orbital fissure.
- Inferiorly and medially it splits to line the fossa and to invest the lacrimal sac.
- Superiorly it forms the pulley of the superior oblique tendon.
- Septae pass from the periorbita to divide the orbital fat into lobules.

## ORBITAL SEPTUM/PALPEBRAL FASCIA

- It is a fibrous sheet that stretches across the entrance of the orbit and is continuous with the periorbita at the rim.
- It is related to the posterior aspect of orbicularis oculi muscle.
- In the upper lid, it unites with the levator aponeurosis and in the lower lid, it fuses with the tarsus and sheath of the inferior rectus.

## BULBAR FASCIA/ TENON'S CAPSULE

- Fibrous sheath surrounding the globe, except the cornea that facilitates eye movement.

## MUSCULAR FASCIA

- Made up by the fusion of the fibrous sheaths of the EOM.
- Surgical space between the periosteum and the muscular fascia—peripheral space.
- Surgical space deep to the muscular fascia, within the muscle cone—central space.

## ORBITAL VESSELS

- Main blood supply to orbit-ophthalmic artery branch of internal carotid artery. It enters through optic foramen.

- Anterior/posterior ethmoid arteries are branches from the ophthalmic artery.
- Parts of inferior orbit are supplied by the infraorbital artery, branch of internal maxillary artery.
- The superior ophthalmic vein and superior branch of inferior ophthalmic vein drain into cavernous sinus through superior orbital fissure.
- Inferior branch of inferior ophthalmic vein communicates with pterygoid plexus by passing through inferior orbital fissure.

## LACRIMAL SYSTEM (*See* Fig. 2.10)

### A. Secretory System

- Basic secretors
  - Goblet cells in conjunctiva
  - Accessory lacrimal glands of subconjunctiva of upper lid
  - Tarsal meibomian glands
- Reflex secretors, lacrimal gland in the lacrimal fossa in the lateral orbit superiorly and anteriorly.

### B. Excretory System

- In each lid there is an opening located medially—punctum
- Punctum leads to canaliculus
- Canaliculus has
  - Vertical component—2 mm in length
  - Horizontal component—8 mm in length
    They joint together to form common canal that empties into lacrimal sac.
- Lacrimal sac is situated in lacrimal fossa situated in anterior part of medial orbital wall
- Lacrimal sac empties into nasolacrimal duct
- Canaliculi and sac are lined with stratified squamous epithelium.

### REFERENCES AND FURTHER READING

1. Stammberger H. Endoscopic endonasal surgery. Concepts in treatment of recurring rhinosinusitis. Part I. Anatomic and pathophysiologic considerations. Otolaryngol, Head and neck surgery 1986;94, 143–155.
2. Hollinshead WH. The head and neck. In: Hollinshead WH. Anatomy for Surgeons. 2nd ed., vol. 1. New York: Harper and Row, 1968.

3.  Myerson. The natural orifice of maxillary sinus, Anatomical studies. *Archives of Otolaryngology*, 1932; Vol. 5, pp. 80–91.

4.  Van Alyea, OE. The Ostium Maxillary anatomic study of its surgical accessibility, *Archives of Otolaryngology*, 1936; Vol. 24, pp. 553–559.

5.  Scheaffer JP. Paranasal sinuses, nasolacrimal passage ways and olfactory organ in Man. Philadelphia. Blakiston, 1920.

6.  **Neivert** H. Surgical anatomy of the maxillary sinus. Laryngoscope 1930; 40:1–4.

7.  Renn, WH and Rhoton, AL Microsurgical anatomy of the sellar region. *The J. Neurosurg.*, 1975; 43:288–98.

8.  Fuji, K; Chambers, A and Rhoton, J. Neurosurgical relationships of the sphenoid sinus: A microsurgical study. *J Neurosurg*, 1979; 50:31–9.

9.  Maniscalco JE, Habal MB. Microanatomy of the optic canal. J Neurosurgery 1978.

10. F Meloni, R Mini, S Rovasio, F Stomeo and GP Tetani. Anatomic variations of surgical importance in ethmoid labyrinth and sphenoid sinus. A study of radiological anatomy, Surgical and radiological anatomy, 1992; Vol. 14; pp. 65–70.

11. Tetani G, Simonet G, Solvini U, et al. Computed Tomography of ethmoid labyrinth and adjacent structure. Normal anatomy and most common variants. Ann Otolaryngology, 1987; 96: 239–250.

12. Van Alyea OE. Nasal sinuses, an anatomical and clinical consideration. 2nd edition, Baltimore (MD) William Wilkins, 1951.

13. Naumann H. Pathologische Anatomie der Chronischen Rhinitis und Sinusitis. In: Proceedings VIII International Congress of Otorhinolaryngology. Amsterdam: Excerpta Medica; 1965. p. 80.

14. Kennedy DW, Zinreich SJ, Rosenbaum AE, Johns ME. Functional endoscopic sinus surgery. Theory and diagnostic evaluation. Arch Otolaryngol 1985;111:576–82.

15. Hollinshead WH. Anatomy for Surgeons, 2nd ed. Vol. 1. The Head and Neck. New York: Harper and Row, 1968.

16. Kasper KA. Nasofrontal connections: a study of one hundred consecutive dissections. Arch Otolaryngol, 1936;23:322–43.

17. Zuckerkandl E: Die Untere Siebbeinmuschel (mittelere nosenmuschel) normal and pathological, Bd1, Bd2 Wein and Leipzeg 1993.

18. Kozlov VS: Anatomical of the endonasal opening of the cells of the ethmoid labyrinth, Vestn Otorhinolaryngology 1975;37,76–9.

19. Rontal E, Rontal M, Guilford FT. Surgical anatomy of the orbit. Ann Otol (1979); 88: 382–386. 20.

20. A Leunig, B Sommer, CS Betz, F Sommer. Surgical anatomy of the frontal recess—is there a benefit in multiplanar CT-reconstruction? Rhinology, 2008; 46, 188–194.

21. Peter J Wormald. Anatomy, three-dimensional reconstruction and surgical technique, 2nd edition, Thieme medical publication, 2002.

22. Benjt JP, Cuilty-Siller C, Kuhn FH. The frontal cell as a cause of frontal sinus obstruction. Am J Rhinol, 1994; 8:185–191.

23. Bent JP, Cuilty-Siller C, Kuhn FA: The frontal cell as a cause of frontal sinus obstruction; Laryngoscope, 1996; 106:1119–25.

24. Keros P: On the practical value of difference in the level of lamina cribrosa of the ethmoid. J Laryngol Rhinol Otol. 1962; 41:808–13

# 2

# Physiology of the Nose and Paranasal Sinuses

## Functions of the Nasal Cavity

- Nasal respiration
- Protection of the lower respiratory tract
- Filtration
- Airconditioning of inspired air (temperature and humidity regulation)
- Mucociliary function
- Sneeze reflex
- Olfaction
- Vocal resonance
- Outlet to the lacrimal secretions

### NASAL RESPIRATION

The contribution of the nose to the airflow in the respiratory tract is of considerable importance. 50% of the total resistance is contributed by the nasal cavities. Man is an obligatory nasal breather for the first 6 months of life. 85% of the adults are nose breathers and only resort to an oral or oronasal route under demanding situation such as exercise or in pathological conditions. It has been estimated that an adult inspires up to 10,000 liters of air daily (Kerr, 1997).

Inspiratory air currents pass vertically up through the anterior nares at a rate of 2 to 3 m/s. The flow converges to a laminar pattern at a velocity of 12 to 18 m/s at the narrowest point, i.e. the nasal valve after which the flow becomes horizontal. Laminar flow is important for cleaning and conditioning of the air. Most of the air conditioning occurs along the middle meatus and the floor of the nose, but eddying occurs in olfactory area (Fig. 2.1a and b).

Expiratory air currents are most turbulent, with air flowing through the nasal cavity, sweeping inspired air out of the olfactory region. The expiratory flow produces eddies in the region of the middle meatus. The sinuses are ventilated only in the expiratory

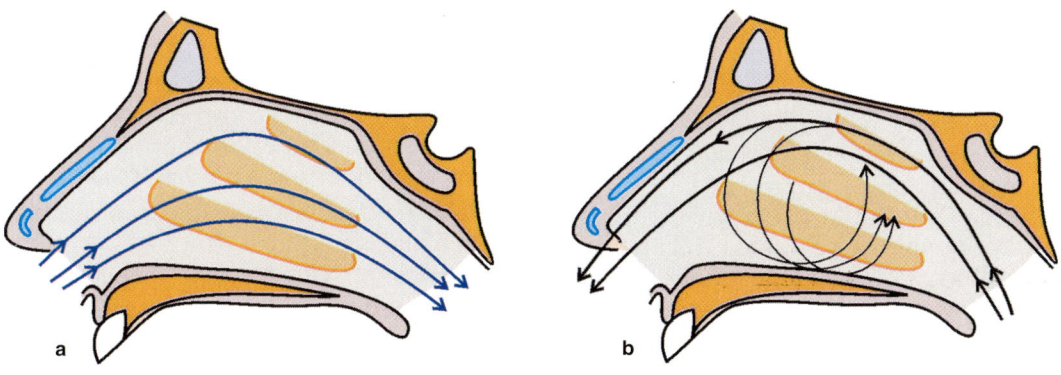

**Fig. 2.1:** Diagram showing inspiratory and expiratory phases of nasal airflow

phase by air that has been pre-treated by the respiratory mucosa and are relatively sterile. The uncinate process probably protects the sinuses by diverting the inspired air that is rich in allergens and bacteriae (Nayak *et al.*, 2001). Figure 2.2 shows the inspiratory and expiratory flow that may get affected by the removal of uncinate process.

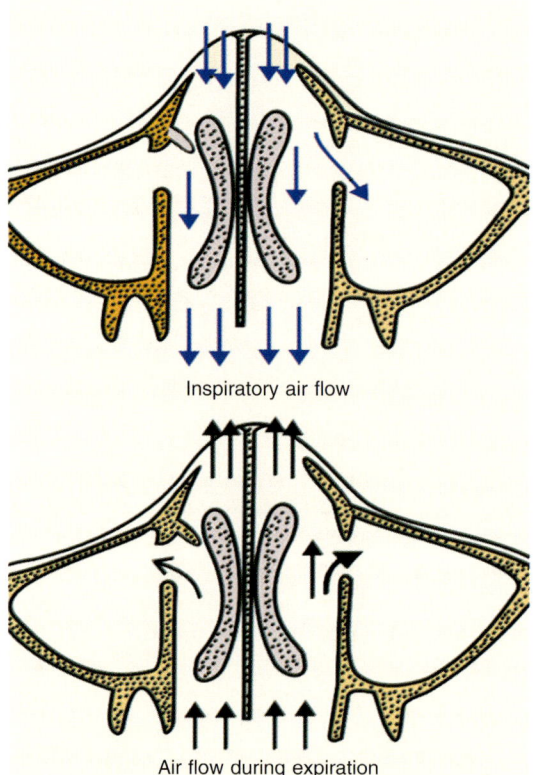

Inspiratory air flow

Air flow during expiration

**Fig. 2.2:** Showing ventilatory mechanism of paranasal sinuses with or without uncinate process preservation (Nayak *et al.*, 2001)

**Nasal airway resistance:** The nasal vestibule is the first component of nasal resistance. The nasal vestibule is composed of compliant walls that are liable to collapse from the negative pressures generated during inspiration (Kerr, 1997). The vestibule has been termed the external nasal valve. Vestibule contributes to one-third of the nasal airway resistance. The valve region is formed slightly posterior to the posterior edge of the lower lateral cartilage and the nasal septum contributes most of the remaining two-thirds of the resistance. The internal nasal valve is the narrowest part of the nasal cavity responsible for controlling the nasal airway resistance and is situated between the cartilaginous nasal septum and lower border of upper lateral cartilage (ULC).

Inferior and middle turbinate contain erectile tissue; the anterior end of inferior turbinate has a major effect on nasal resistance and it functions as an internal nasal valve (Fig. 2.3)

Changes in the nasal resistance are primarily the result of a vascular response and erectile tissue controlled by autonomic nervous system, mainly the sympathetic system. This determines the state of engorgement of the erectile tissue.

### Factors Affecting the Nasal Resistance

a. **Age:** Maximum resistance is found in infancy and it reduces as the age advances

b. **Nasal cycle:**

*Definition:* A physiological cycle of spontaneous reciprocating nasal congestion and decongestion alternating between the two nasal cavities. This was first described by Kayser in 1895 and is probably controlled by respiratory areas in the brainstem closely associated with respiratory activity. The duration of the cycle varies from 2 to 7 hrs. It is absent in laryngectomies and tracheostomised patients.

c. **Exercise:** With increase in exercise the nasal resistance decreases probably due to increase in the sympathetic action on the erectile tissue.

d. **Respiration:** Resistance is slightly lower during inspiration compared to that during expiration. Hyperventilation results in vasodilatation and a rise in resistance.

e. **Posture:** Change of posture leads to change in nasal resistance due to alteration in jugular venous pressure.

f. **Nasal reflexes:** Sneezing can influence the nasal resistance. Sneezing results from a number of mild mechanical and chemical stimuli to the nasal mucosa and is associated

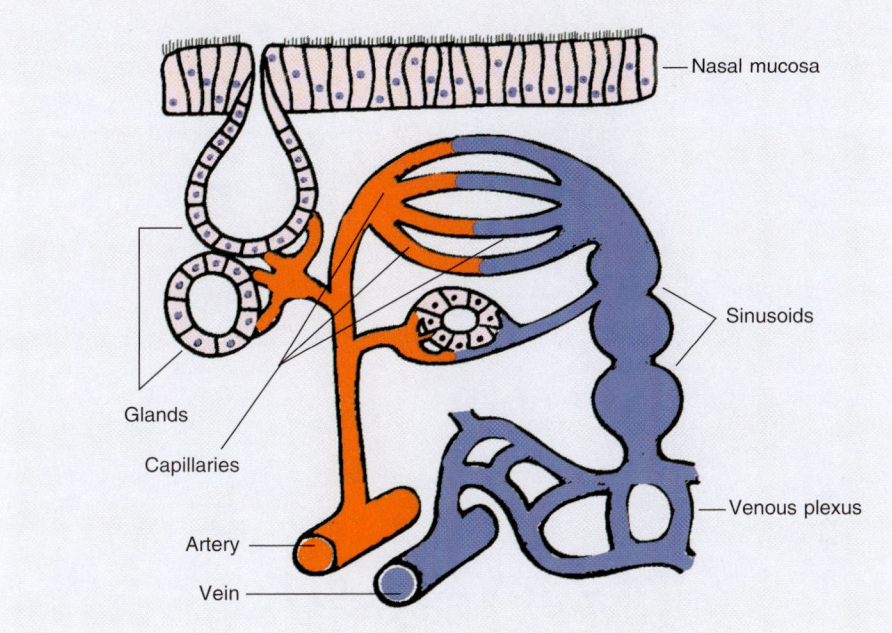

**Fig. 2.3:** Subepithelial erectile tissue of nasal cavity

with increased secretion and congestion. The trigeminal nerve, respiratory muscles and the autonomic nervous system usually mediate this.

g. **Skin and air temperature:** Atmospheric air can affect the skin temperature, which reflexly alters the nasal mucosal blood flow as part of the thermoregulatory mechanism. Cool inspired air can cause congestion and increased resistance.

h. **Emotional and psychological response:** This causes autonomic imbalance and alteration in the nasal resistance by regulating the erectile tissue.

## Protection of the Lower Respiratory Tract

### Filtration

Vibrissae in the nasal vestibule prevent the large particles in the inspired air to pass through the nasal cavity.

### Air-conditioning of the Inspired Air (Fig. 2.4)

The temperature and humidity of the inspired air is regulated by the nasal mucosa. The blood flow of the nasal cavity is from the posterior to anterior direction as shown in Fig. 2.4, which is opposite to the flow of inspired air.

This mechanism is applied in refrigeration industry and is called countercurrent mechanism. This allows the inspired air to be humidified as it comes in contact with the mucous blanket, which also traps the dust particles. The humidification of the inspired air occurs from the evaporation of mucous blanket. The countercurrent effect also allows heating of the inspired air that gets pretreated in the nasal chamber. This air-conditioning function is controlled by the autonomic nervous system.

### Mucociliary Function

Mucociliary clearance is one of the major functions of the nasal epithelium. Respiratory mucosa is coated by a thin layer of mucous secretions called mucous blanket, which helps in cleaning the fine particulate matters that are trapped in it during the inspiratory phase and also helps the cilia to function smoothly to

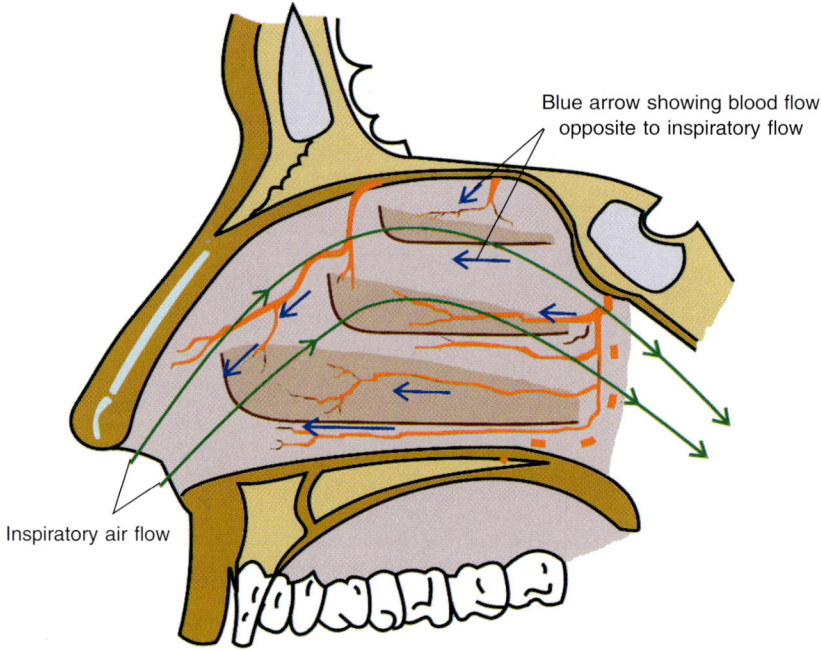

**Fig. 2.4:** The countercurrent mechanism of the air-conditioning function of the nose. Blue arrows show the direction of the blood supply and green arrows showing the direction of the inspiratory airflow

facilitate proper mucociliary clearance. It consists of superficial thick mucous layer (gel) and deep thin periciliary layer (sol) (Fig. 2.5).

The mucous secreting glands and goblet cells of the nasal and sinus mucosa secrete the mucous. The mucous is rich in lysozymes, an important enzyme that initiates bacterial destruction. In addition, it contains secretory IgA, which neutralizes allergens and bacterial toxins (Fig. 2.6).

The cilia of the respiratory epithelium beat in a specific manner and direction and propel the mucous blanket towards the pharynx, where it is swallowed. The cilia are composed

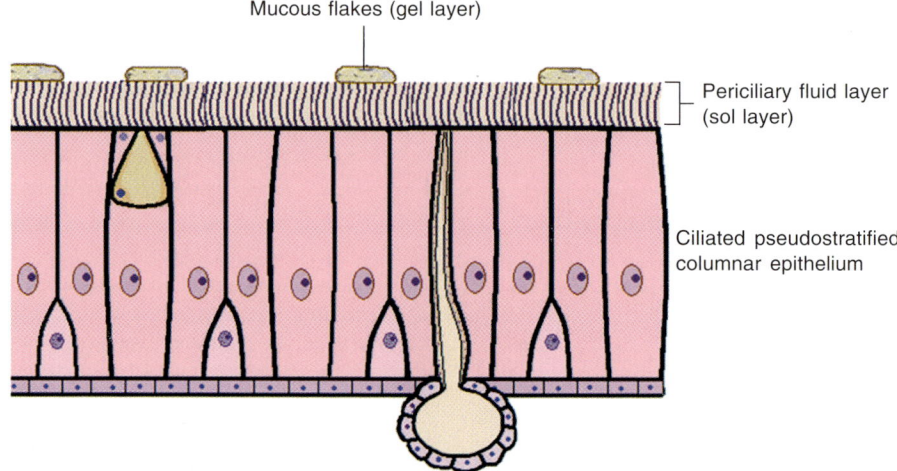

**Fig. 2.5:** Mucous blanket function

contains ATPase responsible for ciliary motility (movement) (Fig. 2.7).

## Nasal Reflex Function and Protection

Clinical observation suggests the existence of poorly characterised reflex pathway between upper and lower respiratory pathway. Sneezing is also a protective function in response to irritants and harmful stimuli.

## Vocal Resonance

The nasal cavities and the sinuses add nasal tone to the articulated voice by acting as resonators. Nasal speech (rhinolalia) results due to nasal or nasopharyngeal obstruction (rhinolalia clausa) or due to abnormal communication between the oral and nasal cavities as in cleft palate and palatal paralysis (rhinolalia aperta).

## Olfaction

It is defined as a mechanism by which the smell is perceived. The olfactory area of the nasal cavity as described earlier is responsible for this function of the nasal cavity. The main functions of olfaction are

- Regulation of the food intake and perception of flavor and palatability
- Regulation of reproductive behavior (more developed in lower animals)
- Protective function: Detection of the noxious and toxic substances.

## Mechanism of Olfaction

The mechanisms by which mammals discriminate a vast array of diverse odors are poorly understood. Olfactory receptors situated in the upper part of the nasal cavity above the level of the superior turbinate sense the odorant particles in the inspired air. Each olfactory receptor neuron has 8–20 cilia that are whip-like extensions 30–200 microns in length. The olfactory cilia are the sites where molecular reception with the odorant occurs and sensory transduction (i.e. transmission) starts. The amount of inspired air reaching this area depends on the nasal anatomy and pathological abnormalities. Sniffing increases the availability of inspired air into the

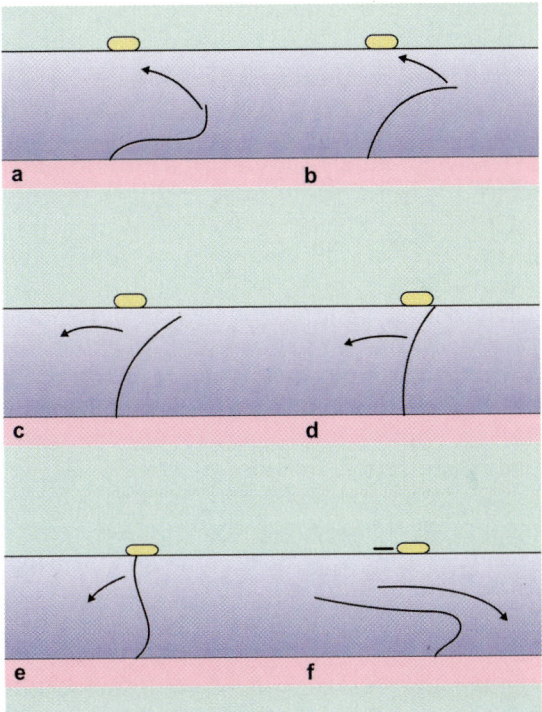

**Fig. 2.6:** Ciliary beat in stages. a. Initiation of beat of cilia. b, c, d, e. Propelling of cilia making the mucous blanket to move. f. Recovery stage

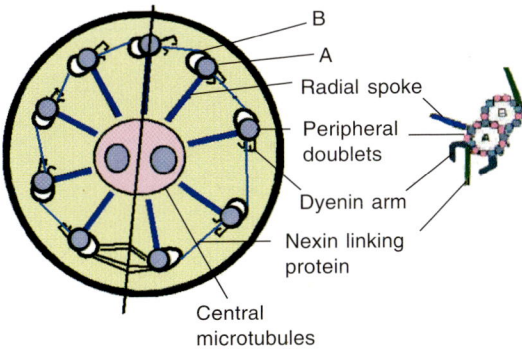

**Fig. 2.7:** The structures of cilia

of multistructural axonema which are composed of nine doublets of peripheral microtubules and two single central microtubules (9+2 pattern). Among the paired microtubules one (A) contains two dyenin arms (outer and inner) extending towards the other microtubules (B) the dyenin arm olfactory area. The regulation of the olfactory system is mainly achieved by the olfactory mechanism, which consists of the olfactory epithelium and its central connections and to some extent by the non-olfactory receptors of the V, VII, IX and X cranial nerves. The Vth cranial nerve perceives odor up to 30%.

## OLFACTORY PATHWAY (Figs 2.8 and 2.9)

### Mechanism of Odor Perception

Many theories exist to explain the mechanism of odor perception. Among them the Lock and Key concept of chemical recognition is widely held. Perception depends on the interaction of the odorant molecules with highly specialized and highly specific olfactory receptor sites in the olfactory cell membrane. The electrical impulse thus generated is transmitted to the higher centers. The odor particles have to cross the mucus to reach the receptor cells, which necessitates it to be water soluble to some extent, but lipid solubility, will enhance interaction with the plasma membrane. Because of the pigments like carotenoids which

are found in the Bowman's glands, a role similar to that of retina has been proposed.

Olfaction is the dominant sensory modality for most animals and chemosensory communication is particularly well developed in many mammals. Our understanding of this form of communication has grown rapidly over the last 10 years since the identification of the first olfactory receptor genes. The subsequent cloning of genes for rodent vomeronasal receptors, which are important in pheromone detection, has revealed an unexpected diversity of around 250 receptors belonging to two structurally different classes. Recent studies using genetically modified mice and electrophysiological recordings have highlighted the complexities of chemosensory communication via the vomeronasal system and the role of this system in handling information about sex and genetic identity. Although the vomeronasal organ is often regarded as only a pheromone detector, evidence is emerging that suggests it might respond to a much broader variety of chemo signals (Flow chart 2.1).

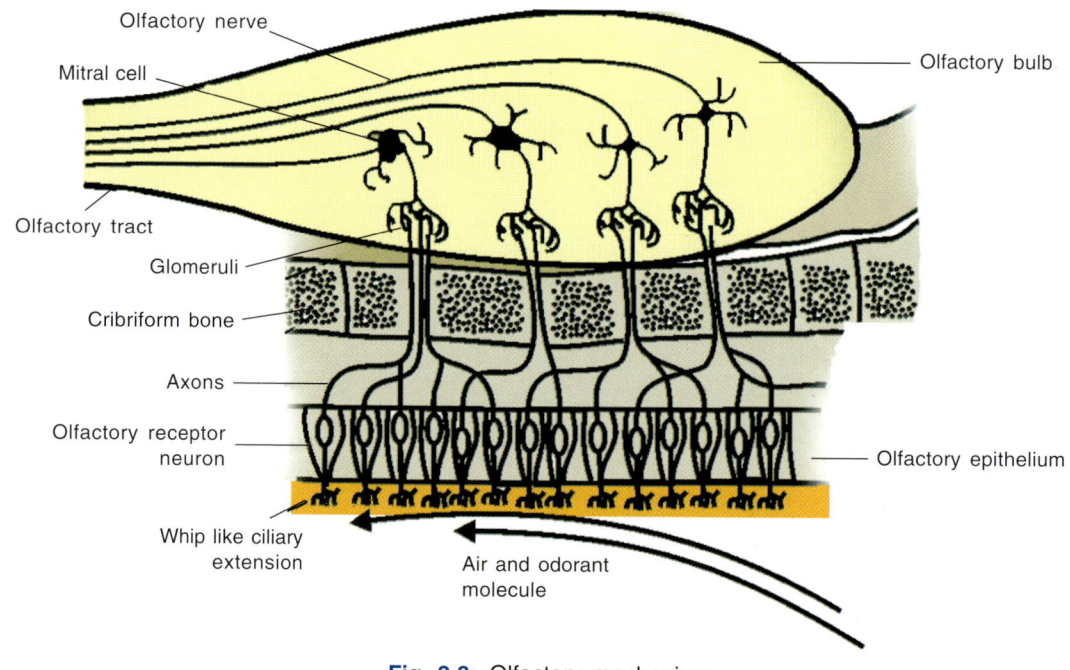

**Fig. 2.8:** Olfactory mechanism

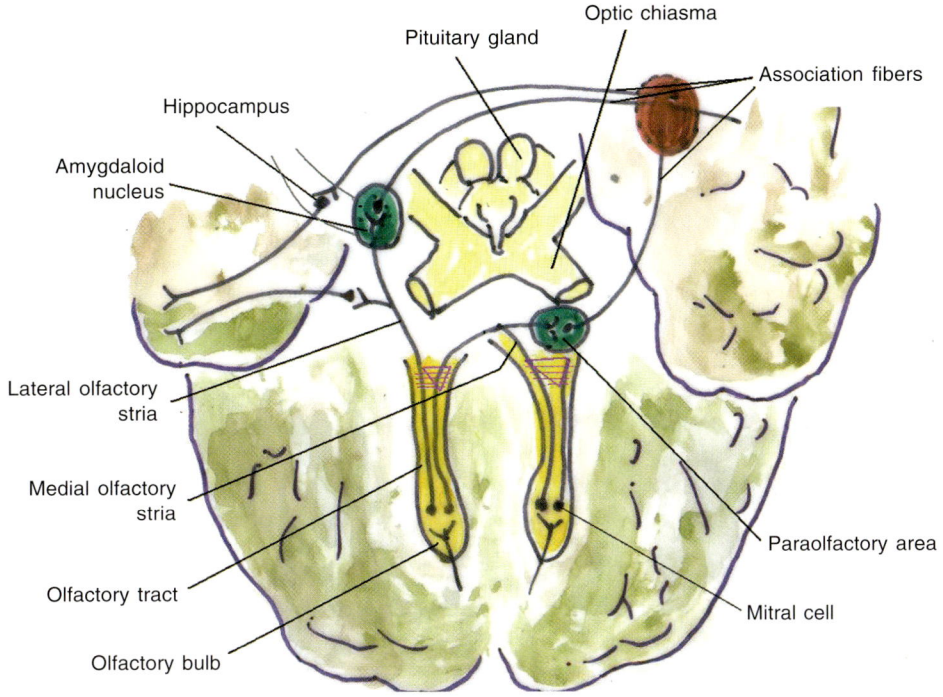

**Fig. 2.9:** Olfactory pathway

**Flow chart 2.1:** Olfactory pathway

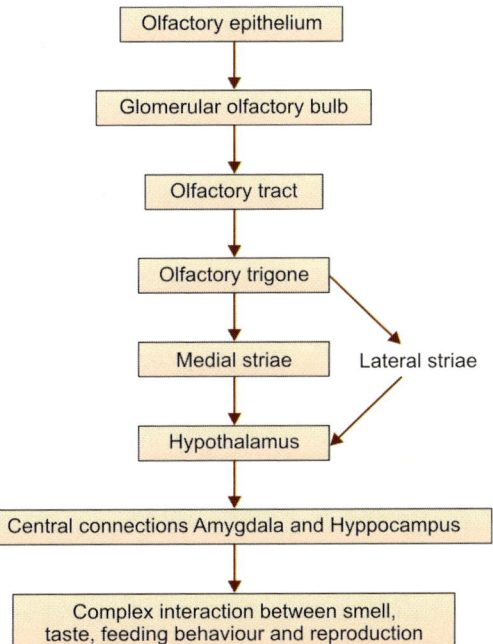

*Outlet for Lacrimation Secretion*

The nasolacrimal duct drains into the inferior meatus. Blockage of this duct can lead to epiphora. Inflammatory conditions of the nose and sinuses like sinusitis and rhinitis, malignancy of the nose and paranasal sinuses can cause obstruction to the lacrimal apparatus and epiphora.

The lacrimal drainage system consists of upper and lower punctum which are situated in the medial aspect of respective eyelids. The puncta leads to the respective vertical and then to horizontal canaliculus. The upper and lower canaliculus joins to form a common canaliculus. The common canaliculus enters the lacrimal sac through the valve of Rosenmuller. This valve of mucosal flap prevents reflux obstruction of common canaliculus that can cause epiphora. The lacrimal sac funnels to form the nasolacrimal duct which opens into the inferior meatus (Fig. 2.10).

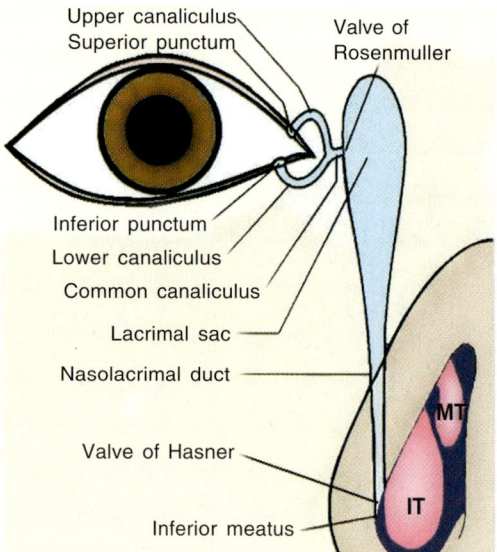

**Fig. 2.10:** The drainage of lacrimal secretions to inferior meatus (IT-inferior turbinate, MT-middle turbinate)

About 70% of lacrimal secretions drain through the lower punctum, while 30% drain through the upper punctum to the lacrimal sac. Chronic rhinitis and sinusitis can cause inflammatory disease of lacrimal apparatus leading to obstruction of nasolacrimal duct.

Endoscopic dacryocystorhinostomy is an effective surgical approach to treat this problem.

## Functions of the Paranasal Sinuses

The function of the paranasal sinuses has been a controversial subject since the time of Galen. Eight hypotheses have received particular attention:

1. They lighten the bones of the skull;
2. Improve the resonance of voice;
3. Humidify and warm the inspired air;
4. Increase the area of olfactory membrane;
5. Serve as shock absorbers in mechanical impacts;
6. Act as thermal insulators of the brain;
7. Promote facial growth and architecture; and
8. Persist as evolutionary relics or faults.

Scrutiny of these hypotheses shows that none has a scientific basis (Gluck 1991). The most important function probably is the mucociliary clearance.

*Mucociliary clearance:* The sinuses act as a constant source of sterile mucous blanket, which is essential to replace the contaminated secretions in the nasal cavity. Secretory mucosa and unobstructed mucociliary transport are absolutely essential for the normal respiratory and olfactory function of the nose and sinuses. Development in nasal endoscopy has revealed more information about the sinus mucociliary clearance activity and in the pathogenesis of sinusitis. Anatomical abnormalities in the nasal cavity especially in the middle meatus can obstruct the outlet of the paranasal sinuses causing persistent inflammatory disease in the sinuses. Mucociliary clearance is described in detail in Chapter 3. The discovery within the paranasal sinuses of the production of nitric oxide (NO) has altered the traditional explanations of sinus physiology. Nitric oxide may be regarded as an "aerocrine" hormone that is produced in the nose and sinuses and the role of NO in the sinuses is likely to enhance local host defense mechanisms via direct inhibition of pathogen growth and stimulation of mucociliary activity (Lundberg 2008).

## REFERENCES AND FURTHER READING

1. Nayak DR, Balakrishnan R and Murthy KD. "Functional Anatomy of the Uncinate Process And its Role in Endoscopic Sinus Surgery " Indian Journal of Otolaryngology And Head and Neck Surgery, 2001: 53(1):27–31.

2. Nayak DR, Balakrishna R and Murthy KD, "Endoscopic Physiologic Approach to Allergy associated chronic rhinosinusitis a preliminary study ENT Journal 2001: 80(6):392–403.

3. Kerr P, Millar T, Buckle P, Kryger M. The importance of nasal resistance in obstructive sleep apnea syndrome. J Otolaryngol 1992;21:189–195.

4. Kerr A, ed. Rhinology. In: Scott-Brown's Otolaryngology. 6th ed. Oxford: Butterworth-Heinemann; 1997.

5. Beauchamp, GK and Yamazaki, K. Chemical signalling in mice. Biochem. Soc. Trans, 2003; 31, 147–151.

6. Doty, RL. Mammalian pheromones: fact or fantasy? In Handbook of Olfaction and Gustation. Doty, RL ed. (Marcel Dekker Inc, 2003).

7. Diseases of ear nose throat, John Jacob Ballenger, 13th edition Philadephia, Lea Feiger 1985.

8. PA Brennan and EB Keverne, Neurobiology. On mammalian pheromones (Current Biology 2004 14:R81).

9. Synopsis of otolaryngology, John Grooves, Roger Gray John Wright and Sons Ltd. 4th and 5th edition.

10. Logan Turners' Diseases of nose, throat, ear by Aruthur Logan Turner and AGD Maraer, Bristol: Wright 1988.

11. Stammberger H: Endoscopic endonasal surgery. Concepts in treatment of recurring rhinosinusitis. Part I. Anatomic and pathophysiologic considerations. Otolaryngol-Head and neck surgery 94, 143–155.

12. Kayser R Die exakte Messung der Luftdurchgängigkeit der Nase. *Arch Laryngol Rhinol* 1895; 3: 101–120.

13. Gluck U. The physiological significance of paranasal sinuses in man: speculations for 1800 years. Schweiz med Wochemschr,1991 Jun 22;121(25):925–31.

14. Lundberg JO, Nitric oxide and the paranasal sinuses. Anat Rec (Hoboken) 2008 Nov;291(11):1479–84.

# 3

# Pathophysiology of
# Chronic Sinusitis

## Definition of Sinusitis

Inflammation of the mucosa of one or more paranasal sinuses where the mucociliary clearance function is affected as a result of anatomical or pathological abnormalities can lead to blockage of the sinus ostia.

Depending on the site of involvement, it can be described as:

- Frontal sinusitis
- Maxillary sinusitis
- Ethmoidal sinusitis
- Sphenoidal sinusitis
- *Pansinusitis:* All sinuses are involved which could be unilateral or bilateral.

In the past, sinusitis was addressed individually with respect to site. The etiopathogenesis, clinical features, investigations and treatment were individualistic. More emphasis was given to maxillary sinus as the most common site of infection.

With clear understanding of osteomeatal complex anatomy and its role in the pathogenesis of chronic sinusitis and with the availability of nasal endoscope and CT imaging for study of sinus pathology, the concept of sinus pathology and its treatment has changed rapidly. The intimate relationship of the sinus system to the nasal cavity and also that of upper and lower respiratory tracts, the role of osteomeatal complex and middle meatus in the etiopathology of chronic infection of the major sinuses has been better understood and changed the treatment policy. Conventional procedures like intranasal antrostomy, Caldwell-Luc operation, etc. have

become almost obsolete and are reserved only for irreversible disease. Present treatment is directed at the disease causation than the result. The osteomeatal disease is endoscopically dealt by functional endoscopic sinus surgery and the physiological sinusotomies are created for better drainage of major sinuses. For example: middle meatal antrostomy for treatment of maxillary sinusitis, frontal recess clearance for frontal sinusitis, etc. (Fig. 3.1).

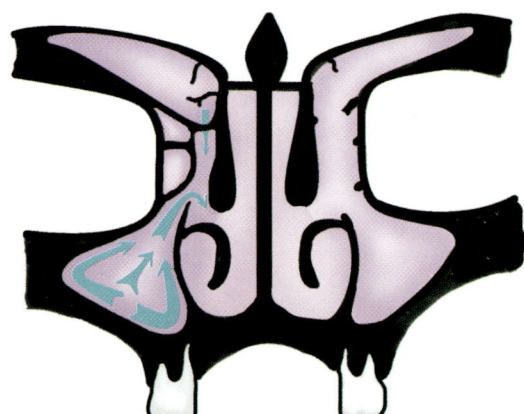

**Fig. 3.1:** Mucociliary clearance before and after endoscopic sinus surgery (after Stammberger)

## Pathophysiology

Normal mucociliary function of nose and sinuses provide a first line defense to the health of the respiratory tract. Failure of normal mucus transport and decreased sinus ventilation are the major factors contributing to the development of sinusitis. Mucosal edema and the anatomic abnormality can

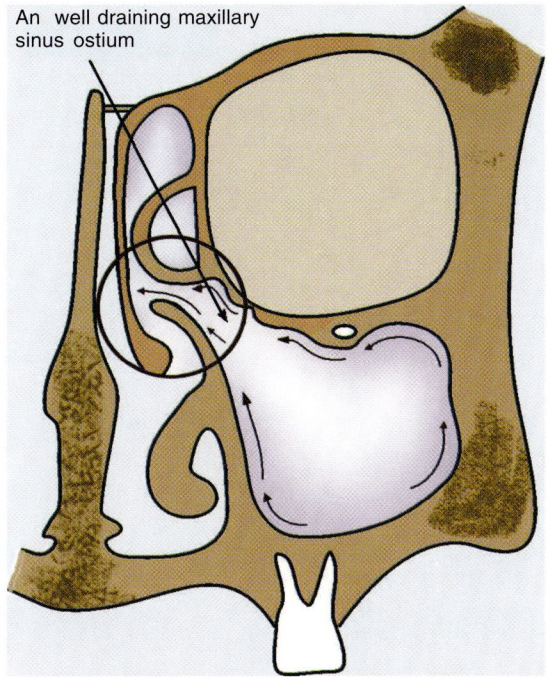

An well draining maxillary sinus ostium

**Fig. 3.2a:** Normal mucociliary clearance

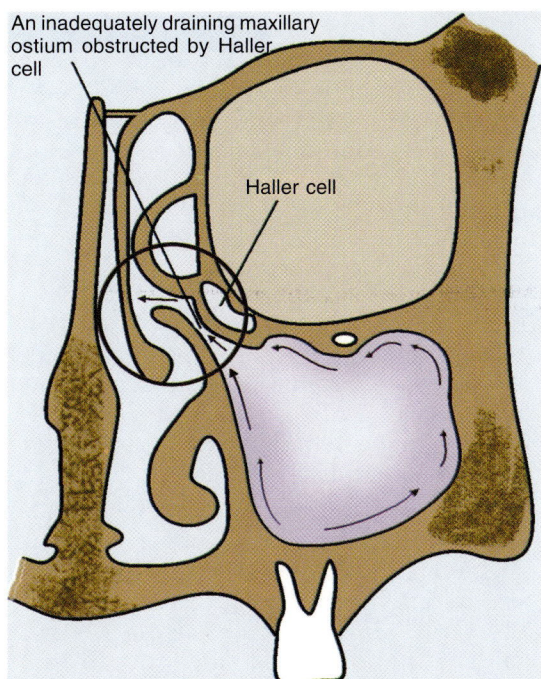

An inadequately draining maxillary ostium obstructed by Haller cell

Haller cell

**Fig. 3.2b:** Normal mucociliary clearance of the maxillary sinus is affected by Haller cell

interfere with drainage of the sinuses as a result of obstruction of the sinus ostium. Figures 3.2a and b show (a) normal mucociliary clearance (b) mucociliary clearance of the maxillary sinus is affected by Haller cell. Better understanding of the mucociliary activity of the paranasal sinuses and the nasal cavity has made the modern rhinologists aspire for a more physiological and hence a functional surgical modality of treatment for chronic and recurring sinusitis. Details of the mucociliary activity is described below to facilitate better understanding of the pathogenesis of chronic sinusitis.

## Mucociliary Activity of Maxillary Sinus

(Fig. 3.3)

The secretions from the maxillary sinus start in a star-like shape from the floor of the sinus along its walls to reach the inner maxillary ostium at the uppermost and posterior corner of the sinus in the lateral nasal wall.

From here, it is actively transported through the ethmoid infundibulum over the

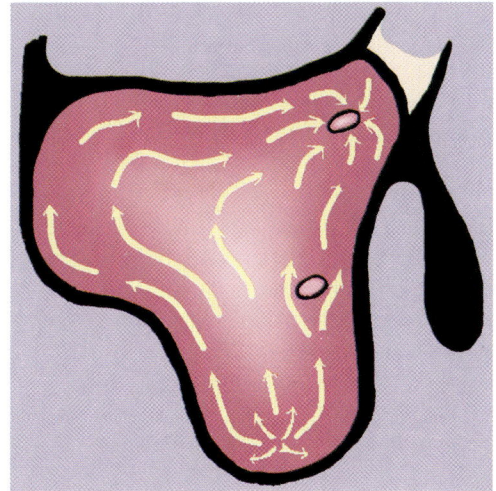

**Fig. 3.3:** Mucociliary activity of maxillary sinus. Note how the mucous stream is bypassing the accessory ostium and moves towards the natural ostium (after Stammberger)

rear margin of uncinate process onto the medial surface of inferior turbinate and then towards the nasopharynx.

The mucous moves along the margin of the ostium towards the natural ostium, when an accessory ostium is present probably guided by gravity. Similarly, a surgically made inferior meatal window fails to actively drain the sinus, but does drain to some extent guided by gravity.

## Mucociliary Activity of the Frontal Sinus
(Fig. 3.4a)

Messerklinger demonstrated an inward transport along the interfrontal septum, along the roof and walls of the sinus laterally, returning to the floor of the sinus and leaving the inner ostium laterally.

Not all the secretions leave the sinus at once. The ethmoidal prechamber to frontal sinus, a certain amount of secretion again joins the inwardly directed pathway and thus enters the sinus again. This retrograde pathway into the sinus helps in spread of infection from the ethmoids into the frontal sinus.

Ethmoidal infundibulum is considered as ethmoid prechamber of maxillary sinus and probably similar retrograde flow exists here also. The frontal sinus drains into the infundibulum, if uncinate process is attached to the skull base superiorly and drains directly into the middle meatus, if the attachment is to the lamina papyracea.

From the frontal recess, the secretion passes to the ethmoid infundibulum, joins the secretion from maxillary sinus and then it is transported towards the nasopharynx. Drainage of frontal sinus can be affected by obstruction to the frontal recess (Fig. 3.4b). The mucociliary drainage of the sphenoid sinus depends on the site of the ostium and usually it has a spiral transportation. The ethmoidal cells may have a direct or a spiral drainage pathway depending on the site of the ostium into their respective meatuses.

## Mucociliary Activity of Lateral Wall of Nasal Cavity (Fig. 3.5)

Two streams of mucous pass on the lateral wall nasal cavity. The first from the anterior

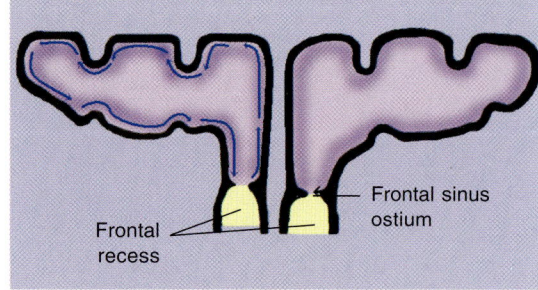

**Fig. 3.4a:** Mucociliary activity of the frontal sinus

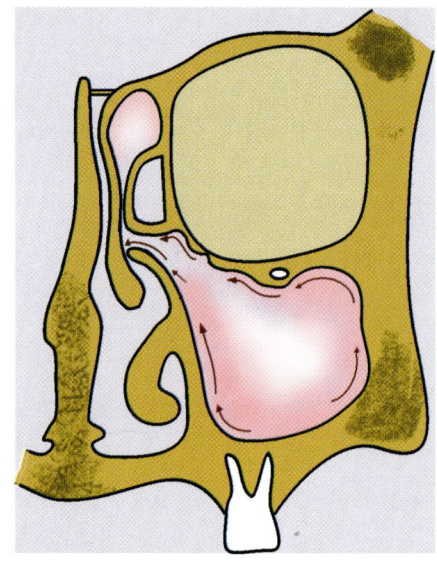

**Fig. 3.4b:** Mucociliary drainage of frontal recess and maxillary sinus is affected by septoturbinal compression

group sinuses onto the medial surface of inferior turbinate via infundibulum and then anterior and inferior to the tubal orifice in the nasopharynx. The second stream from the posterior group of sinuses passes above the middle turbinate and then posterior and superior to the tubal orifice. Thus in relation to the tubal orifice, two streams are supratubal and infratubal streams of mucous from anterior and posterior groups of sinuses respectively (Fig. 3.5).

Acute or chronic nasal and sinus inflammation causes alteration in the normal and well-defined pathway. As illustrated the following may occur (Fig. 3.6).

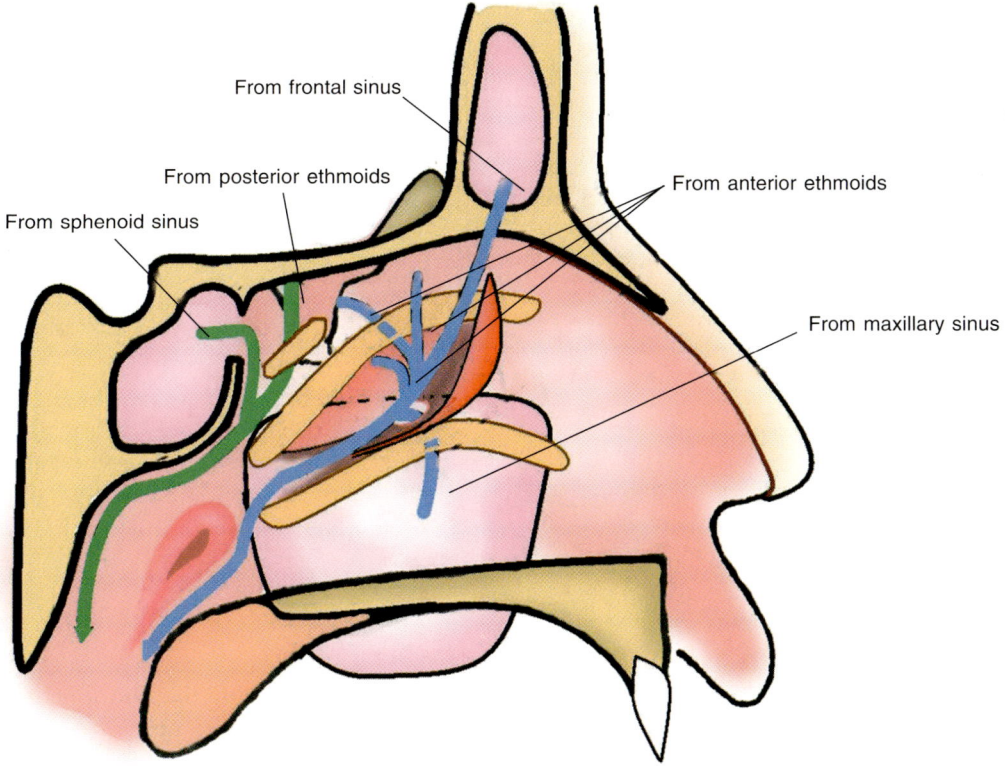

**Fig. 3.5:** Mucociliary activity of lateral wall of nasal cavity

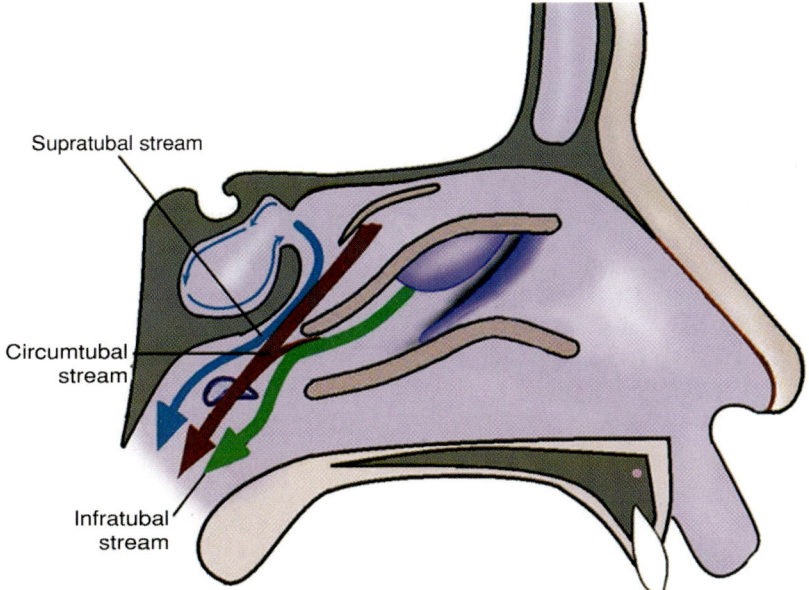

**Fig. 3.6:** Alteration in normal mucociliary pathway associated with sinus inflammation

- The routes can join before reaching the tubal orifice (Fig. 3.6).
- One or both routes may form whorls around or even in the orifice itself (Fig. 3.6).
- Abnormal secretions may thus move directly over the orifice perse (Fig. 3.6).

Any factor that impedes the physiologic mucociliary clearance and ventilation of the sinuses cause chronic sinusitis.

Unfortunately the sinuses drain into the nasal cavity through a complex micro-architectural pathway through the anterior ethmoid and the middle meatus. This system of fissures and clefts within the anterior ethmoid draining the maxillary and frontal sinuses is called osteomeatal complex and comprises of ethmoid infundibulum, frontal recess and maxillary sinus ostium.

These microchannels can be obstructed by various anatomical and pathological variations, however trivial they may be. Also, the ethmoid sinus because of its topographical situation, is the primary site of deposition of bacterial and allergic particles and thus a primary site of inflammatory disease.

Procter in 1966 said *'The ethmoid sinuses are usually the key to any problem involving the infectious sinusitis.* Infection begins there and persistent infection there is usually the reason for failure of therapy directed at any of the other paranasal sinuses'.

*Thus the ethmoid sinuses and the osteo-meatal complex play a crucial role in patho-genesis by*

1. Obstruction to the drainage pathway can occur due to anatomical variations that are very common in anterior ethmoid and as it is the primary site of inflammatory disease, pathological variations are also very common.
2. Acting as the reservoir of infection.
3. Reinfects the dependent sinuses by means of retrograde flow.

Most infections of the PNS are rhinogenic. Other sources of primary infection are dental, blood borne or traumatic. Whatever the source of infection is, in chronic sinusitis, even though the primary source of infection is cured, the ethmoid sinus continues to harbour infection.

*Rhinogenic cause of infection is either due to:*

- Primary infection of the nasal and sinus mucosa by bacteria, viruses, etc.
- Secondary to chronic rhinitis due to allergy, vasomotor response or obstructive patho-logies of nasal cavity like DNS, polyps, tumour, synechiae, foreign bodies, etc.

Thus in most of the cases, chronic sinusitis is actually a chronic rhinosinusitis. Thus the treatment of this condition should also eliminate the rhinogenicity.

*The osteomeatal obstruction can occur either due to* anatomical variations or patho-logical variations in the osteomeatal complex.

## ANATOMICAL VARIATIONS

### Variations of Uncinate Process

#### Medially Turned Uncinate Process

The free posterior margin may be deflected medially, narrowing the middle meatus, thus obstructing the drainage pathway. This may also contact the middle concha.

#### Laterally Turned Uncinate Process

This narrows the ethmoid infundibulum and if occurs anteriorly, blocks the frontal recess.

#### Anteriorly Bent Uncinate Process

This may contact the middle turbinate. It narrows the middle meatus and may appear as an additional turbinate. Such a situation is referred to as double middle turbinate.

**Uncinate bulla** (pneumatised uncinate process)

This can narrow the ethmoid infundi-bulum, frontal recess or the middle meatus.

#### Fracture of the Uncinate Process

This could be either traumatic or iatrogenic, due to infracture of the inferior turbinate as in procedures like INA, Caldwell-Luc, etc. This infracture produces lateral movement of uncinate process, thus obstructing the ethmoid infundibulum.

## Variations of Middle Turbinate

### Paradoxically Turned Middle Turbinate

Has its convexity towards lateral nasal wall thus narrowing the middle meatus. This is often found bilaterally and in the anterior aspect of middle meatus. In severe cases it may compress all the delicate structures in the lateral middle meatal wall.

### Concha bullosa (pneumatised middle turbinate)

The pneumatisation makes the middle turbinate bulky, narrowing the airway, middle meatus, frontal recess, ethmoid infundibulum and hiatus semilunaris. Also, the cell may get infected aggravating its pathogenicity.

Three patterns of pneumatisation have been described with respect to their position in the MT (Bolger *et al* 1991).

1. In the inferior or bulbous segment (31.2%)
2. In the superior or lamellar segment (46.2%)
3. Extensive pneumatisation of both (15.7%)

The types 1 and 3 are said to be more significant.

### Overpneumatized Bulla

This makes bulla more bulky, and may compress the uncinate process associated with narrowing of the infundibulum, frontal recess, obstructing the hiatus semilunaris. It may also fill in the middle meatus, touching the middle turbinate and thus narrowing the middle meatus. Infected bullar cells aggravate the situation by producing mucosal thickening on the surface of the bulla.

The space above and posterior to the bulla is called sinus lateralis. This is another narrow, hidden space. Disease from bulla may reach posterior ethmoid through this space.

### Haller's Cells

These are anterior ethmoid cells, pneumatising the floor of the orbit, precisely in the region above and lateral to the maxillary sinus ostium and infundibulum. This can narrow the ostium or the infundibulum mechanically by virtue of either dimension of the cell or due to disease within it. These cells are implicated as possible etiologic factor in recurrent maxillary sinusitis (Fig. 3.2b).

### Overpneumatized Agger Nasi Cells

Agger cells which are the anterior most cells of anterior ethmoids are situated anterior and superior to the insertion of the middle turbinate to lateral nasal wall.

This may be over pneumatised usually bilaterally and usually starting from the frontal recess area.

This may narrow the frontal recess and also the middle meatus at the insertion of middle turbinate, leaving only a tiny fissure. When diseased, it may completely block the above.

**Nasal septal spur:** Bony spur of nasal septum can occupy and obstruct the middle meatus.

## Pathological Variations

Pathological variations like mucosal edema or hyperplasia, polypi, etc. could be due to persistent infection or allergy. These commonly occur in the anterior ethmoids as they are primary sites of inflammation. In addition, the anatomical variations which are very common in anterior ethmoids predispose to formation of polypi by creating narrow pathways for passage of air (Bernoulli's phenomenon). Also, contact areas may cause polyp growth by the local liberation of neuropeptides such as substance P, which is also a factor in mediating pain. Thus small polypi are frequently found within the hiatus, infundibulum, frontal recess and for that matter in any area of mucosal contact like between over pneumatised bulla and middle turbinate.

The infundibular diseases are reflected on the medial surface of uncinate process as congested, thickened mucosa, with or without polypi and perforations in uncinate process discharging mucopus. The disease in the bullar cells is reflected on the surface of bulla with similar findings. In diseased frontal recess, in addition to the anatomical variations like prominent agger nasi, congestion and mucopus discharge may be found in this area endoscopically.

Synechiae formed in the middle meatus either due to previous surgery or trauma from nasal packing, nasotracheal or nasogastric intubation, etc. can cause OMC disease.

Thick viscid mucous can plug the intricate passages of anterior ethmoid. Ciliary motility disorders like Kartagener's syndrome, mucoviscidosis, polycystic disease, etc. can impair mucociliary activity causing chronic sinusitis.

Thus a functional endoscopic sinus surgery should aim at:

1. Elimination of the ethmoid reservoir of infection by anterior ethmoidectomy.
2. Creation of physiological sinusotomies for mucociliary guided drainage.

By achieving the above (as in Fig. 3.1), it has been shown that even the mucosal disease

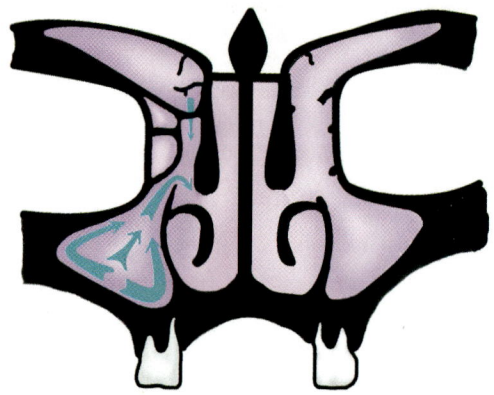

**Fig. 3.7:** Mucociliary clearance in pre- and postoperative endoscopic sinus surgery (after Stammberger)

in the major sinuses which was considered irreversible, reverts to normal.

The pathogenesis is summarised in Flow chart 3.1.

**Flow chart 3.1:** Pathogenesis of chronic sinusitis

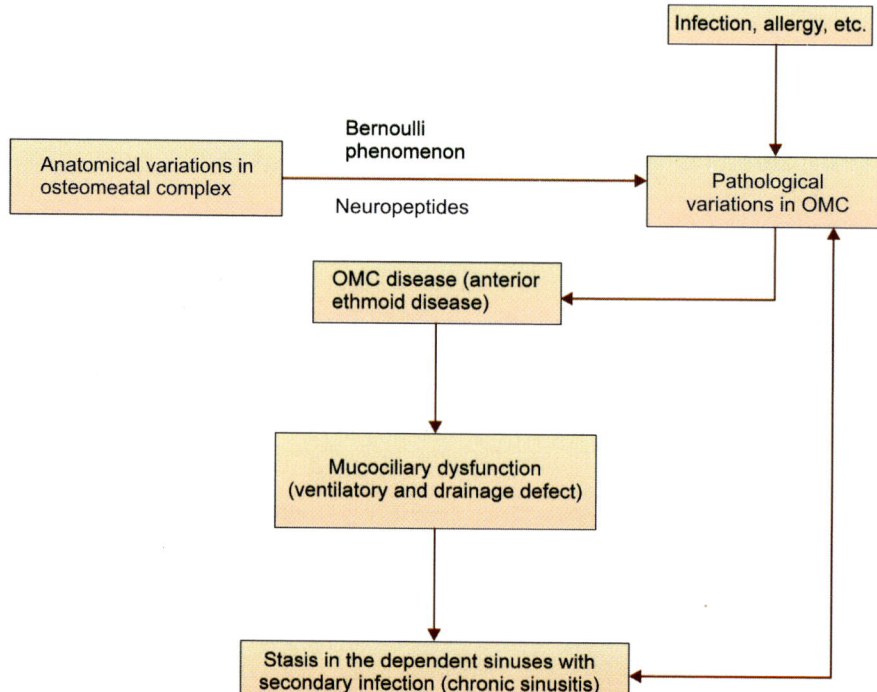

## REFERENCES AND FURTHER READING

1.  Stammberger H. Nasal and paranasal sinus endoscopy. A diagnostic and surgical approach to recurrent sinusitis. Endoscopy, 18, Nov. 86, pp 211–256.

2.  Kennedy *et al.* Endoscopic middle meatal antrostomy. Theory, technique and patency. Laryngoscope. 1987. Vol. 97, Supp., pp 143.

3.  Stammberger H. An endoscopic study of tubal function and the diseased ethmoid sinus. Arch. Otorhinol. Laryngol. 1986, 243. pp 254–259.

4.  Kennedy et al. Functional endoscopic sinus surgery. Part 1. Theory and diagnostic evaluation. Arch otolaryngol Vol. III. Sept. 1985. pp 576–582. Part II. Surgical technique. Arch otolaryngol Vol. Ill, Oct. 1985, pp 643–649.

5.  Stammberger H. Endoscopic endonasal surgery. Concepts in treatment of recurring rhinosinusitis. Part I. Anatomic and pathophysiologic considerations. Otolaryngol-Head and neck surgery 94, 143–155.

6.  Howard L. Levine. Functional endoscopic sinus surgery. Evaluation, surgery and follow up of 250 patients. Laryngoscope. 100, Jan. 1990, pp 79–84.

7.  Nayak *et al.* Endoscopic physiological approach to nasosinus allergy. Ear Nose Throat Journal, Jan (2001).

8.  Zinreich et al. Paranasal sinus, CT imaging requirements of endoscopic surgery. Radiology 163. 1987, pp 769–775.

9.  Stammberger H. Nasal and paranasal sinus endoscopy. A diagnostic and surgical approach to recurrent sinusitis. Endoscopy 18, Nov. 86, pp 211–256.

10. Stammberger H and Wolf. Headaches and sinus disease : The endoscopic approach. Ann: Otol. Rhinol. Laryngol. 1988. Supp. 134, pp 3–23.

11. Stammberger H. Endoscopic surgery for myeotic and chronic recurring sinusitis. Ann. Otol. Rhinol. Laryngol. 1985, Supp. 94. 101–119.

12. Bolger et al. Paranasal sinus surgery. Anatomic variations and mucosal abnormalities. CT analysis for endoscopic sinus surgery. Laryngoscope, 101, Jan. 1991, pp 56–64.

13. Kerr A, ed. Rhinology. In: Scott-Brown's Otolaryngology. 6th ed. Oxford: Butterworth-Heinemann; 1997.

14. Proctor DF: The nose, paranasal sinus and pharynx, in Walters W (ed), Lewis Walters, practice of surgery, Hagerstown, Maryland, WF Prior, 1966, Vol 4, pp 1–37.

# 4

# Diagnostic Nasal Endoscopy

The nasal telescope is an optical instrument for examining the nose. This examination is known as diagnostic nasal endoscopy. The most important thing is that the hidden areas can be precisely visualised, assessed and effectively treated with the help of telescopes. Diagnostic nasal endoscopy and functional endoscopic sinus surgery are relatively new techniques that have expanded our understanding of sinus physiology and the etiologies of sinus pathology. Diagnosis at an early stage of chronic sinus disease demonstrates that pathological changes are often limited to the osteomeatal complex and the anterior sinus group. Early disease refractory to aggressive medical management usually responds to surgical treatment (Levine 1991).

One of the most revolutionary changes seen in rhinology in the recent past is the use of telescope to visualise the lateral nasal wall pathologies as a cause of recurrent sinusitis and to treat these effectively. Antroscopy and nasal endoscopy help to peep inside maxillary sinus and nose, and provide information which is superior to that obtained by other investigations. Both these can be conveniently performed as an outpatient procedure under local anesthesia.

Narrow, stenotic areas in the anterior ethmoid especially in the vicinity of infundibulum where the frontal and maxillary sinuses drain, are the key areas for detection and cure of infection of the anterior group of paranasal sinuses which is made possible by the use of nasal endoscopy. Nasal cavity findings obtained by nasal endoscopy were more conclusive in the elucidation of diagnosis than those obtained by computer tomography of the paranasal sinus (Duarte et al. 2005).

## Technology

Major technical advances in optics and lighting have produced rigid endoscopes suitable for use in nasal and sinus endoscopies.

Hopkins optical rod lens system has improved upon traditional endoscopes by producing bright and sharp images with a larger viewing angle. Hopkins rod lens system was introduced in 1960. Traditional telescopes employed a group of lenses constituting an objective followed by a succession of relay systems.

In rod lens system, the image is relayed by a succession of rod lens. The traditional systems consisted of a tube of air with thin lens of glass. By contrast the new system may be regarded as a tube of glass with thin lenses of air (Hopkins-Modern urological endoscope).

Advantages of using rod lenses are
1. The total light transmitted is increased by factor $n^2$, where n is the refractive index of glass used for lenses.
2. Mechanically the case and precision of mounting of rod lenses permit a greater diameter to be used for lenses for a given outer diameter of telescopes.
3. The use of efficient, multi-layer, anti-reflection coatings on the surface of lenses contribute notably to the brightness.

The function of endoscopy itself is to render the interior of body cavity observable to the endoscopist exactly as if it were being viewed by him directly.

The nasal endoscope is an optical instru-ment for examining the nasal cavity. This examination is known as diagnostic nasal endoscopy. As the endoscope is between 2.7 and 4.0 mm in diameter, it can be passed easily through the nostril to examine the nasal passages and the sinuses. In 0° nasal endoscopes, the view is straight ahead from the tip of the instrument, whereas in other endoscopes, the view is at an angle from the tip of the endoscope. These angled endoscopes can be used to visualise the remote areas of the nasal cavity and paranasal sinuses. The Hopkins rod-lens system has brought about a revolutionary change in technology of endoscopy (Fig. 4.1).

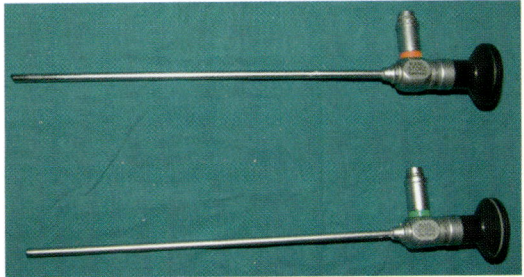

**Fig. 4.1:** Karl Storz 0° and 30° nasal endoscope

In the performance of comprehensive diagnostic nasal endoscopy, the most commonly employed telescopes are the 0° and 30° endoscopes. The instruments are 18 cm long glass rod lenses, with an outside diameter of 4 mm. For special indications like children or in patients with stenotic meati, the 0° and 30° lenses with 2.7 mm outer diameter scopes are used. The telescope with a deflection angle of 70° is helpful in visualising frontal recess.

For routine examination, illumination is provided by Karl Storz 481-C miniature light source, whereas for photo documentation a Karl Storz 610 Xenon light source with built in flash generator is employed.

The video equipment includes a television camera, beam splitter, colour monitor and recorder (Fig. 4.2).

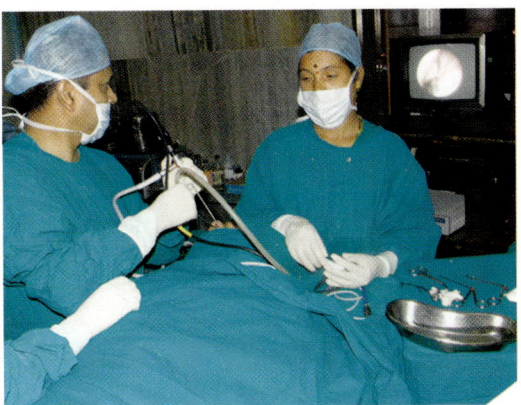

**Fig. 4.2:** Showing video nasal endoscopic assessment before starting functional endoscopic sinus surgery

## Indications for Diagnostic Nasal Endoscopy

Diagnostic nasal endoscopy is an essential investigative modality in the following situations:

1. Patients with gross sinusitis diagnosed clinically to reach a pathological diagnosis (Osteomeatal Complex Disease).
2. In patients with symptoms attributable to sinusitis to confirm diagnosis.
3. In patients whose problems are not clear and in whom there seems to be no overt indication of sinus disease, this group of patients present rewarding challenge for the nasal endoscope (Stammberger 1988).
4. In patients with headaches due to non-sinus disease, to rule out concurrent sinus involvement.
5. In allergic rhinosinusitis for early detection of nasal polyps.
6. In patients with chronic dacryocystitis to visualize the nasolacrimal duct and to rule out any nasal causes.
7. In cases of rhinosinusitis to decide if surgery will be the effective therapy.
8. For postoperative objective evaluation after sinus surgery.
9. For taking nasal swabs for cultures under endoscopic control (Kennedy, 1985).
10. In tubotympanic disease to detect occult sinusitis.

11. In patients with epistaxis to localise bleeding points.
12. To detect small foreign bodies in the nose.
13. To establish if a deflected nasal septum is significant enough to cause the symptoms.
14. To diagnose adenoids and other naso-pharyngeal masses. It has replaced Yanker's nasal speculum to examine nasopharynx.
15. To evaluate eustachian tube orifice.
16. To diagnose chronic nasal diseases like rhinosporidiosis, mycosis, rhinolith, etc.
17. For post maxillectomy evaluation.
18. In pain therapy by blocking the spheno-palatine ganglion.

### Selection of Patients

Diagnostic nasal endoscopy has to be done in a quiescent stage of sinusitis. Patients encoun-tered with acute exacerbation of chronic sinusitis may be put on medical treatment for 7–10 days before embarking on diagnostic nasal endoscopy.

Diagnostic endoscopy can be performed in any age or sex. Nasal endoscopy is a safe, objective and useful means of identifying potentially significant abnormalities in children with nasal obstruction (Kubba and Bingham 2001).

Before doing a nasal endoscopy checking lignocaine sensitivity is a must to avoid catastrophies. Blood pressure estimation will detect hypertensive patients in whom adrenaline should not be used for nasal decogestion.

Other systemic diseases like diabetes-mellitus, tuberculosis, bronchial asthma and bleeding diathesis pose no contraindication to nasal endoscopy. As for apprehensive patients, a gentle reassurance will allay anxiety.

### 1. Equipment

• Nasal endoscopes. Hopkins rod optical system with cold light source and fiber-optic light delivery system provides excellent illumination and optical quality. Endoscopes are available with 0°, 30°, 70°, 90°, 120° angles of view and 2.7 and 4 mm diameter (Fig. 4.1).

• Topical decongestant and anesthetic agent and applicators. 4% xylocaine with 1:100,000 adrenaline.
• Antifog solution
• Suction apparatus and suction cannula

### 2. Position

Supine with head slightly turned towards the examiner who is seated on the right side of the patient (Fig. 4.3).

Gustafson et al. (1989) describes the patient in sitting position, with the examiner sitting opposite, facing him.

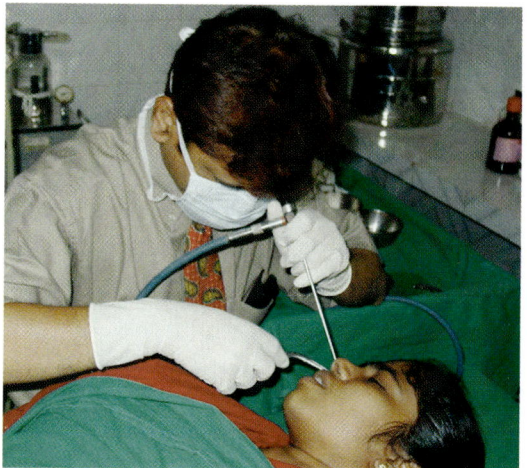

**Fig. 4.3:** Showing outpatient diagnostic nasal endoscopy in progress

### *Anesthesia*

Topical decongestant anesthetic spray (4% lignocaine + 1:100,000 adrenaline) followed by application of the same solution using applicator like cottonoid strips on the floor of nasal cavity, over the inferior turbinates, sphenopalatine foramen area, middle meatus and the anterior aspect of the roof, to block anterior ethmoidal nerve. Applicator is left in position for 10 minutes.

Gustafson et al. (1989) uses phenyl ephrine hydrochloride as decongestant. Huerter (1992) uses mixture of oxymetazoline in 4% ligno-caine in 1:1 ratio. Kennedy uses 5% cocaine on a nasal applicator to the inferolateral surface of the middle turbinate and to other sites, where passage of endoscope may exert slight pressure. In case where significant septal deviation is present, topical cocaine is also applied to the posterior nasal mucosa on the side of convexity.

### 3. Antifog Solution

The scope may be get fogged due to deposition of moisture. Huerter (1992) used antifog solution FRED to prevent fogging. Kennedy says that if telescope lens is touched against clean mucous membrane such as interior end of middle turbinate, is all that is needed to prevent fogging.

In our set up we use savlon solution, and also ask the patient to breath through the mouth to prevent fogging.

### 4. Endoscopy

The endoscope is gently held using both hands. The left hand rests on the patients face and holds the endoscope using thumb and index finger. Right hand holds the eyepiece. Movements are made gently avoiding trauma. It is essential that the instrument is gripped lightly so that the examiner readily detects undue pressure and avoids discomfort. In adult 4 mm. 30° telescope is selected first. This

provides an excellent overall view of nose and nasopharynx (Kennedy 1985).

Huerter (1992) uses 2.7 mm 30° endoscope as it allows good visualization of even narrow noses. Gustafson (1989) uses 4 mm, 0°–30° and 70° for routine examination.

#### I Pass

Along the floor of nasal cavity towards nasopharynx look for:
a. Status of inferior meatus and turbinate should be noted. Hypertrophic turbinates are usually associated with DNS and chronic rhinitis. Turbinates may be atrophied in atrophic rhinitis (Fig. 4.4b).
b. Patency of nasolacrimal duct orifice.
c. Status of INA window, if present and status of antral mucosa, if visualised.
d. Septal spur (Fig. 4.5)
e. Eustachian tube orifice and nasopharyngeal mucosa. Look for stream of mucus, which could be supratubal, infratubal circumtubal or over the orifice (Fig. 4.4a).
f. Dynamic action of tubal orifice may be visualised. Foossor of Rosenmuller is examined.

#### II Pass

After completing examination in the Ist pass, the scope is withdrawn and slide over the medial surface of the middle turbinate. The

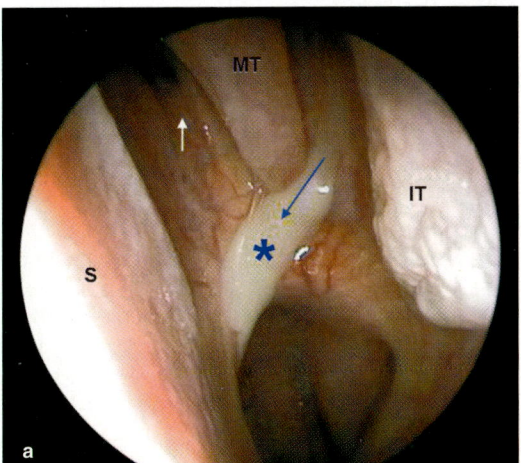 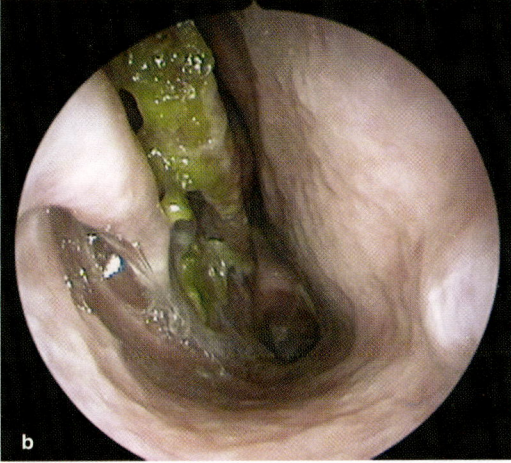

**Fig. 4.4: a.** Thick puralent discharge from left middle meatus seen above the eustachian tube orifice. **b.** Greenish yellow crusts seen in the posterior part of nasal cavity associated with atrophy of the turbinates

scope is further advanced between the middle turbinate and the septum to reach the spheno-ethmoidal recess. Any discharge if present should be noted. Further advancing the scope upwardly in the region will allow the visibility of the sphenoid sinus. Decongestion of this area between the septum and the middle turbinate is very essential for good visualization.

### III Pass

This is the most important pass of the three that evaluates the middle turbinate and the middle meatus. The agger nasi is evaluated at the anterior attachment. Middle meatus is rarely wide enough to admit the telescope anteriorly. It can be frequently inserted into the posterior aspect of middle meatus to inspect bulla, hiatus semilunaris, infundi-bulum, etc. Look for any anatomical variations in the OMC like concha bullosa (Fig. 4.5) medially turned uncinate process (Fig. 4.6), etc.

The pathological variations in the OMC are polyp in the middle meatus (Fig. 4.7), or mucoidal discharge in the middle meatus (Figs 4.5 and 4.8), purulent discharge in the middle meatus (Fig. 4.9). Frontal recess area is visualised to look for any discharge from the frontal recess. Swelling may be seen at the

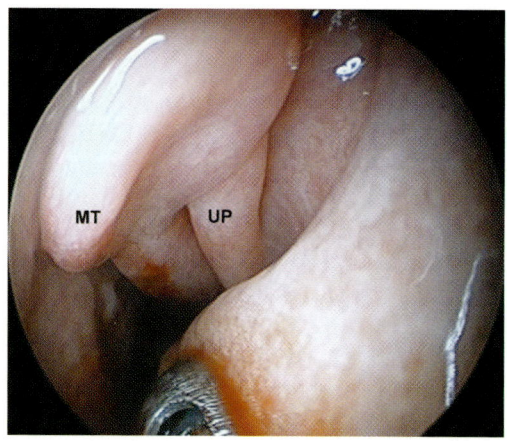

**Fig. 4.6:** Endoscopic picture of a medially turned uncinate process

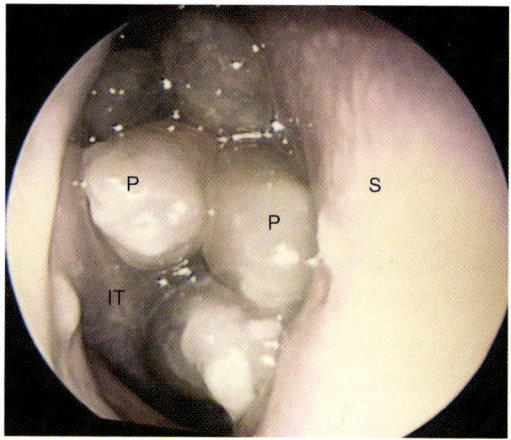

**Fig. 4.7:** Polyps in the middle meatus

attachment of middle turbinate in case of fronto-ethmoidal mucocele.

### Other Methods

Gustafson (1989) uses a different technique. The scope is carefully passed along the floor of the nose while the septum, inferior meatus, inferior turbinate, middle turbinate and nasopharynx are inspected. The telescope is then gently raised to expose the face of sphenoid, the sphenoid ostium and spheno-ethmoid recess. The telescope is then rolled up over the posterior tip of inferior turbinate into the posterior aspect of middle meatus. As the telescope is withdrawn anteriorly, visualize the structures in middle meatus.

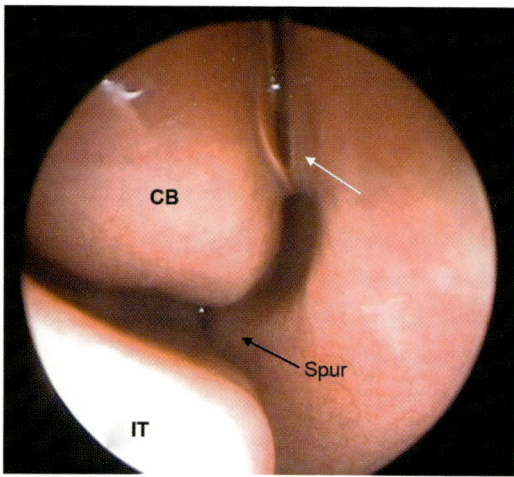

**Fig. 4.5:** Endoscopic picture of left concha bullosa and septal spur. Also note mucoid discharge between septum and middle turbinate seen in a case of allergic rhinosinusitis, from posterior ethmoids (white arrow)

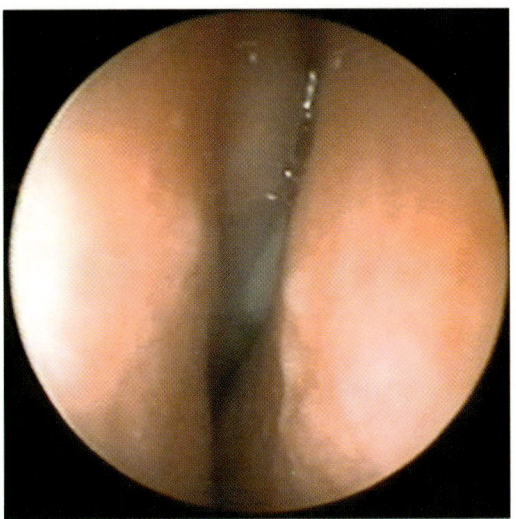

**Fig. 4.8:** Endoscopic picture showing mucoidal discharge in the middle meatus

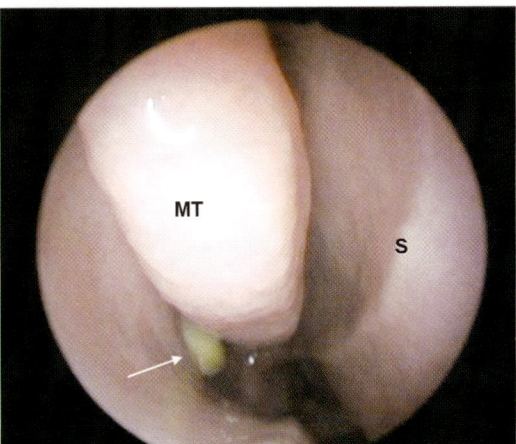

**Fig. 4.9:** Purulent discharge in the middle meatus

The inspection of maxillary sinus mucosa through a postoperative middle on inferior meatal antrostomy is facilitated by angle telescope (70°) of 2.7 mm size.

The endoscope can be passed along the floor of the nasal cavity till the nasopharynx. The scope is withdrawn between the inferior and middle turbinates to evaluate middle meatus. The scope enters the middle meatus in a posterior inferior direction and moved anterosuperiorly to evaluate hiatus semilunaris, bulla ethmoidalis and nasofrontal recess. At this point, the scope is passed medial to the middle turbinate, posterosuperiorly to observe the superior meatus spheno-ethmoidal recess and sphenoid ostium (Huerter 1992).

Kennedy advises gentle medial subluxation of middle turbinate or the use of a cannula placed under middle turbinate to help the introduction of 4 mm, scope in middle meatus.

### Nasal Endoscopy in Children

Performing nasal endoscopy in a child can be a very difficult problem and in many cases, we may have to resort to GA.

Chait *et al*. (1991) has described their technique for successful pediatric examinations.

a. The environment of the examination room should be calm and the approach to the child must be gentle.

b. 2% cocaine solution (instead of 5%) is applied gently to the child's nostril 8–10 sprays are administered. Nasal cottonoids are not used.

c. Cocaine will produce a bitter taste and the child should be forewarned of this.

d. Introduce the scope gently into the nose shielding the light from child's eye.

### Limitations of Nasal Endoscopy

1. Gross septal deviation can make endoscopy difficult and unrewarding.

2. Localized disease within the infundibulum, frontal recess and maxillary sinus ostium is difficult to diagnose.

3. Optical illusory effect due to this, a beginner may find it difficult to orient the anatomy especially when using different optical views.

4. Depth perception is not there because of absence of binocular vision.

5. Gives no information regarding position and status of vital relations of spheno-ethmoids.

6. Exact extent of disease within the spheno-ethmoid is difficult to be made cut.

These limitations can be overcome by CT imaging of OMC.

## REFERENCES AND FURTHER READING

1. Levine SB, Gill AJ, Levinson SR, Coffey TK. Diagnostic nasal endoscopy and functional endoscopic sinus surgery: an update and review of complications. Conn Med. 1991 Oct; 55(10):574–6.

2. Aracely Fernandes Duarte, Rita de Cássia Soler, Francis Zavarezzi Rev Bras. Nasal endoscopy associated with paranasal sinus computerized tomography scan in the diagnosis of chronic nasal obstruction Otorhinolaryngol.V.71, n.3, 361–3, May/June 2005.

3. Stammberger H, Wolf G. Headaches and sinus disease: the endoscopic approach. Ann Otorhinolaryngol 1988 Sept–Oct 134:3.

4. Haytham Kubba and Brian JG Bingham. Endoscopy in the assessment of children with nasal obstruction, Journal of Laryngology and Otology (2001), 115: 380–384 Cambridge University Press.

5. Kennedy DW. Arch Otolaryngol 1985;111:643–98.

6. Gustafson RO, Kern EB. Office endoscopy when, why, what, and how. Otolaryngol Clin North Am. 1989 Aug; 22(4):683–9.

7. Huerter JV. Functional endoscopic sinus surgery and allergy. Otolaryngol Clin North Am. 1992;25(1):231–238.

8. Duarte AF *et al.* Nasal endoscopy associated with paranasal sinus computer tomography in the diagnosis of chronic sinusitis. Rev Bras Otorhinolaringology V71, N-3, p 361–363, May/June 2005.

9. Chait DH & Lotz WK, Successful pediatric examination using nasoendoscopy, Laryngoscope, 1991 101 (9): 1016–1018.

# 5

# Indications for Endoscopic Surgery of the Nose and PNS

Functional endoscopic sinus surgery is a relatively minimally invasive technique and the goal of this procedure is to restore sinus ventilation and normal function (Stammberger 1991). It is the most successful in patients who have recurrent acute or chronic infective sinusitis. Initially the indication for endoscopic sinus surgery was confined to the management of chronic sinusitis refractory to medical treatment, but over the years the indications for endonasal endoscopic surgery have extended to encompass a wide variety of diseases other than just chronic sinusitis. The effectiveness of standard surgical techniques for inflammatory diseases of nasal and paranasal sinuses has been well established for more than a century. With the recent popularization of endoscopic sinus surgery, however, many of these techniques are now considered radical (Friedman 1989).

Endoscopic sinus surgery is most commonly performed for inflammatory and infectious sinus disease. Tabulated below are all the indications and extended indications for endoscopic nasal and sinus surgery.

## Indications for Endoscopic Sinus Surgery

1. Chronic sinusitis (Figs 5.1 and 5.2)
2. Recurrent sinusitis
3. Fungal sinusitis
4. Nasal polyposis
5. Excision of concha bullosa
6. Partial turbinectomy
7. Allergic fungal sinusitis
8. Epistaxis
9. Synechiae release
10. Endoscopic bipolar cauterization of inferior turbinates
11. Sinus mucoceles

## Extended Indications for Endoscopic Sinus Surgery

1. Mucoceles
2. Pyoceles
3. Cerebrospinal fluid leak
4. Optic nerve decompression
5. Orbital cellulitis/abscess
6. Foreign bodies from the paranasal sinuses
7. Osteoma nasal cavity/PNS
8. Meningoceles/meningoencephalocele
9. Contact headache/neuralgia

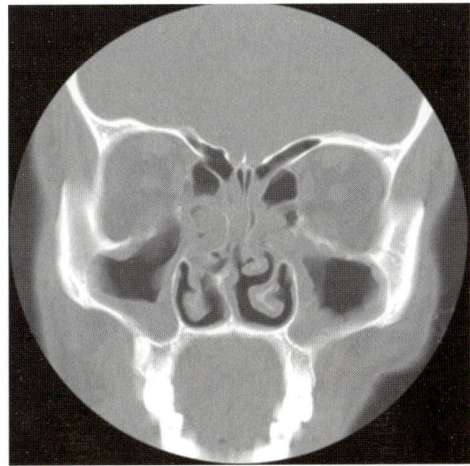

**Fig. 5.1:** Chronic pan-sinusitis associated with bilateral osteomeatal complex disease

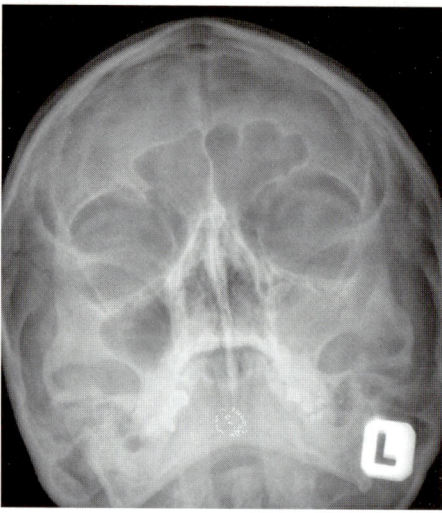

**Fig. 5.2:** X-ray PNS (Water's view) showing left chronic maxillary sinus opacity with thickened mucosa of the right maxillary sinus and haziness of right frontal sinus in a patient with chronic sinusitis

## Indications for Endonasal Endoscopic Surgery

1. Endoscopic septo-turbinoplasty.
2. Endoscopic medial maxillectomy, craniofacial resection, etc and skull base surgery.
3. Atrophic rhinitis.
4. Dacryocystorhinostomy.
5. Pituitary tumors (endoscopic hypophysectomy).

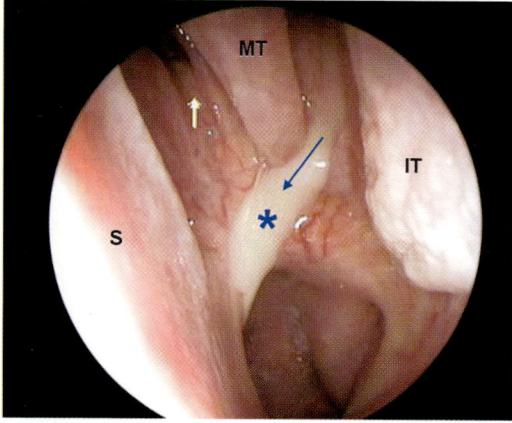

**Fig. 5.3:** Muco-purulent discharge from left middle meatus moving towards nasopharynx

6. Adenoidectomy
7. Congenital choanal atresia
8. Rhinosporidiosis
9. Vidian neurectomy
10. Nasopharynx biopsy
11. Inverted papilloma
12. Sphenopalatine ganglion block
13. Meningoceles/meningoencephalocele
14. Impacted foreign bodies in the nose

Chronic sinusitis usually involves the anterior ethmoids and maxillary sinuses. Pansinusitis, involvement of all the sinuses, almost always including the posterior ethmoidal cells with or without the sphenoid and frontal sinuses.

Recurrent sinusitis is defined as periodic episodes of acute sinusitis with complete clearance of disease in between. As a result of frequent infection and the disease confined to the anterior ethmoids, it is mandatory to undergo endoscopic surgery especially when the disease interferes with our daily routine work.

Fungal sinusitis is usually associated with immunocompromised patients and can be treated successfully through endoscopic sinus surgery. Clearance of the disease is possible under direct endoscopic vision and repeated inspection of the FESS cavity. Allergic fungal sinusitis can be associated with polypoidal changes and polyp formation in the middle meatus (Figs 5.4 and 5.7).

Nasal polyposis can be surgically removed by endoscopic surgery. Polyps seen in the younger age group can avoid extensive procedures like external ethmoidectomy which leave a scar, thus causing psychological trauma. For antrochoanal polyp, Caldwell-Luc operation is a morbid procedure if the facial skeletal growth and dentition is not complete (Fig. 5.8).

Intranasal glioma can be safely excised through endoscopic approach (Fig. 5.9).

Persistent nasal obstruction due to concha bullosa or extensive hypertrophied inferior turbinates can be resected endoscopically to relieve the obstruction and also fashioned to prevent a roomy cavity. Synechiae formation

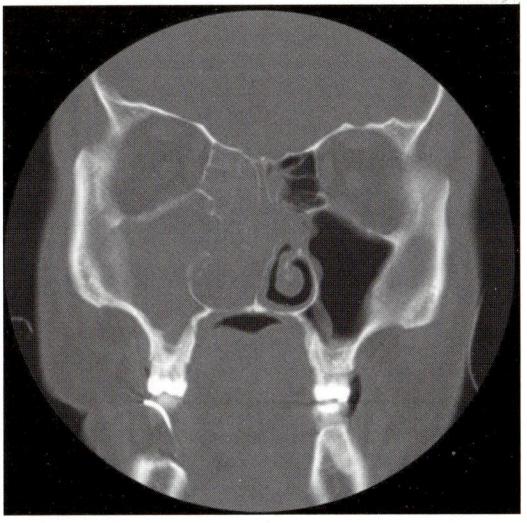

**Fig. 5.4:** Coronal CT scan of osteomeatal complex showing gross involvement of left maxillary sinus and ethmoids in a case of allergic fungal sinusitis

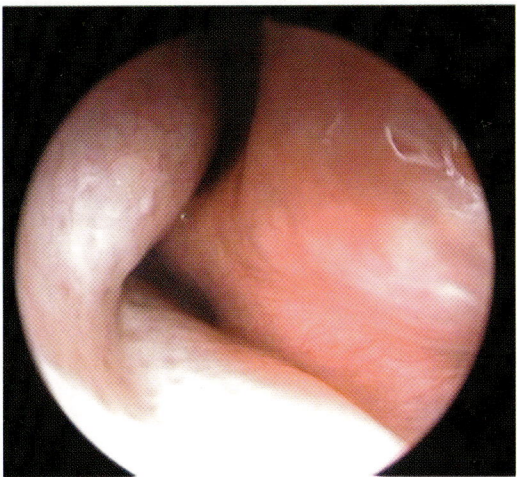

**Fig. 5.6:** Video endoscopic photograph showing septal spur in contact with lateral wall

after extensive intranasal polypectomy or multiple nasal surgeries can be relieved. A dental wax plate can be inserted to prevent further adhesions (Fig. 5.10).

Posterior nasal bleeds occur from the sphenopalatine vessels, which can be easily identified and cauterized. Hypertrophied, edematous inferior turbinate particularly the posterior part which may occlude the posterior choana can be endoscopically cauterized by a bipolar cautery, or reduced by laser.

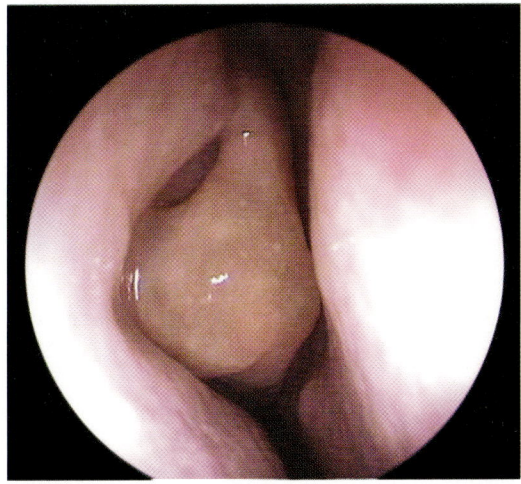

**Fig. 5.7:** Video endoscopic photograph showing polypoidal middle turbinate

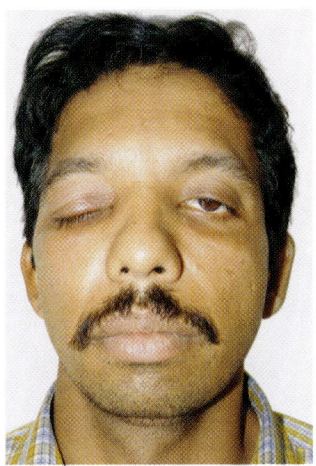

**Fig. 5.5:** Right orbital cellulitis

Frontal and ethmoidal mucoceles are more common than maxillary and sphenoidal mucoceles. Mucoceles and pyoceles can be treated successfully by endoscopic sinus surgery thus preventing a radical external approach and maintaining the normal physiological features and drainage pathway of the sinus.

Cerebrospinal fluid leak is commonly caused by trauma and leak into the floor of the nasal cavity through the cribriform plate.

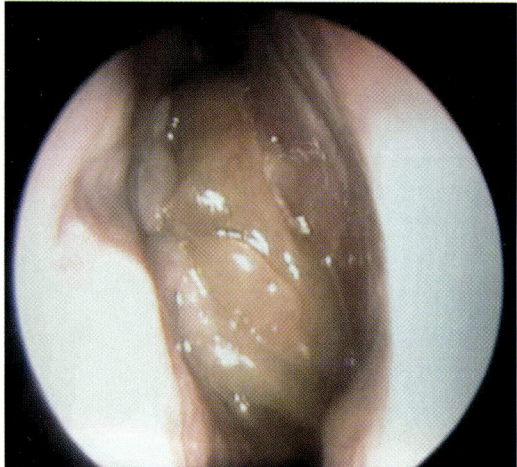

**Fig. 5.8:** Video endoscopic photograph showing ethmoidal polyposis

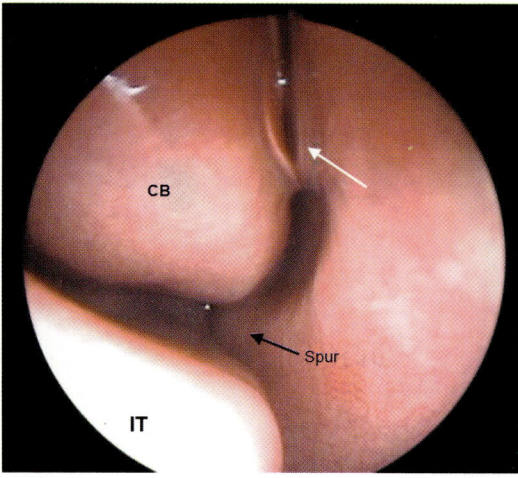

**Fig. 5.10:** Endoscopic picture showing septal spur, concha bullosa and clear discharge from superior meatus

sphenoid sinus surgery. The lateral wall of the sphenoid sinus is exposed and drilled, thus relieving the compression on the optic nerve.

Foreign bodies in the paranasal sinuses are rare, more so in the sphenoethmoidal complex. Penetrating wound caused by a ricocheted air gun pellet lodged the posterior ethmoid labyrinth has been successfully removed by endoscopic intranasal ethmo-idectomy. Nasal foreign bodies can be shown endoscopically.

Endoscopic dacryocystorhinostomy is performed to connect the lacrimal sac directly to the nasal cavity when there is an obstruction either in the sac or in the nasolacrimal duct (*see* Chapter 14). Osteomas are bony tumors commonly seen in the frontal sinus. Endoscopically one can reduce or resect these osteomas with a drill.

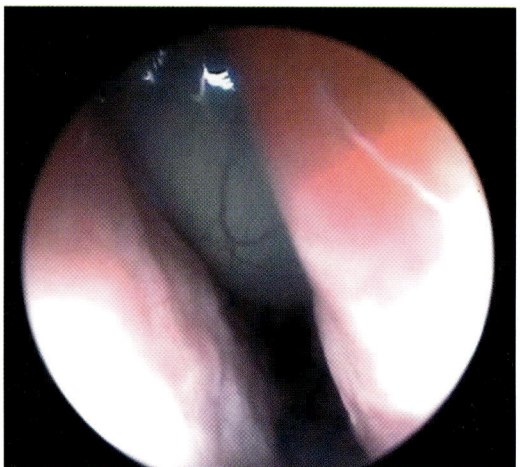

**Fig. 5.9:** Video endoscopic photograph showing intranasal glioma

Endoscopic repair is possible by using a temporalis fascia muscle graft and placing it at the leaking site. The graft is further supported by abdominal fat and gel foam.

Orbital decompression has its indications. By endoscopically removing the lamina papyracea and floor of the orbit, the orbit can be decompressed providing excellent results. Orbital cellulitis and abscess can be drained by opening the lamina papyracea and incising the orbital periosteum. Even optic nerve decompression can be achieved by endoscopic

Sphenopalatine ganglion block as a primary mode of pain therapy is clinically used for a variety of disorders of the head and facial regions. Endoscopically the sphenopalatine foramen is identified between the posterior ends of the middle and superior turbinates. The sphenopalatine ganglion is located lateral to the sphenopalatine foramen. A long acting local anesthetic (0.25% Bupivacaine) is administered repeatedly. Vidian neurectomy has been endoscopically performed with promising results.

Congenital choanal atresia can be corrected by endoscopic intranasal or endoscopic sublabial transnasal approach. A portex naso-tracheal tube stent is left *in situ* for a period of two to three weeks.

Postoperative cavities following medial maxillectomy or craniofacial resection are inspected regularly for any infection or recurrence by nasal endoscopes. Post-operative assessment of the nasal mucosa for atrophic rhinitis in modified Young's opera-tion is possible by endoscopes, thus helping to determine the optimum time for reversal of Young's procedure.

Using a 30° endoscope the entire naso-pharynx may be examined. In addition to the eustachian tube orifice, presence of any abnormal mass or early nasopharyngeal malignancy can be taken for biopsies. Recurrent epistaxis due to rhinosporidiosis can be located in the hidden areas of the nose such as inferior meatus, middle meatus, roof of the nasal cavity and the roof of the nasopharynx. It can be visualized, cauterized from its base and removed in Toto endo-scopically.

Recently endoscopic approach has been adopted to perform medial maxillectomy and anterior skull base surgery for removal of benign tumors like inverted papilloma, haemangioma, glioma, angiofibroma, etc. of the nasal cavity, paranasal sinuses and nasopharynx. Malignant tumors of the nasal cavity and paranasal sinuses without gross intracranial involvement can be removed by exclusive endoscopic/endoscopic assisted minimally invasive surgery depending on the extent of the disease in selected cases.[17] Dural defect can be repaired with fascia lata graft and septal flap (Hadad flap).

Pituitary tumors can be approached endoscopically through trans sphenoidal route. Meningocele and Meningo-encephalocele can be excised endoscopically. CSF leaks commonly associated with these surgeries can be repaired at the same sitting using the temporalis fascia, septal cartilage along with abdominal fat.

Endoscopic adenoidectomy has become popular nowadays because of minimal risk of

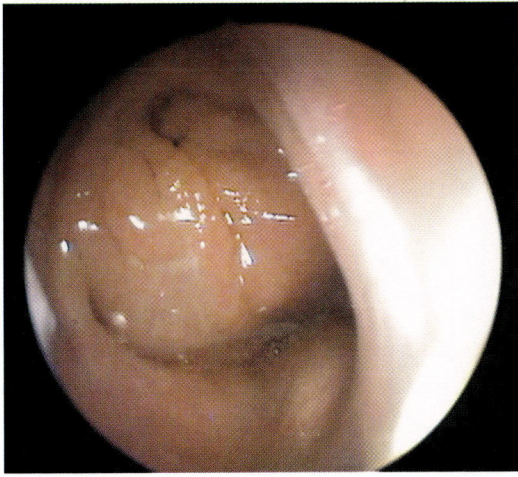

**Fig. 5.11:** Video endoscopic photograph showing adenoid hypertrophy occluding the postnasal space

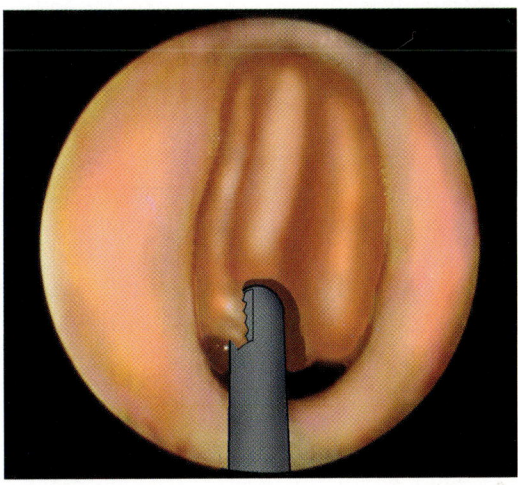

**Fig. 5.12:** Micro-debridor assisted endoscopic adenoidectomy in progress

complications. Nayak *et al.* first described endoscopic adenoidectomy in case of Scheie's syndrome and later described superiority of endoscopic adenoidectomy over traditional adenoidectomy (Figs 5.11 and 5.12).

Endoscopic septoplasty is performed to precisely correct only the deviated part of the septum, so that the endoscope can pass freely into the nasal cavity, thus enabling a functional endoscopic sinus surgery to be preformed. Nayak *et al.* (1998, 2001) described various endoscopic abnormalities of nasal septum and the associated lateral wall pathology and there management by ultra-conservative septo-turbinoplasty.

## REFERENCES AND FURTHER READING

1. Stammberger H. Functional endoscopic sinus surgery: The Messerklinger technique. Philadelphia: Decker, 1991:283.

2. Wigand ME. Endoscopic surgery of the paranasal sinuses and anterior skull base. New York: Thieme Medical Publishers, 1990:1–2.

3. Kennedy DW, Zinreich SJ, Rosenbaum AE, Johns ME. Functional endoscopic sinus surgery. Theory and diagnostic evaluation. Arch Otolaryngol 1985; 111:576–82.

4. Kennedy DW. Functional endoscopic sinus surgery. Technique. Arch Otolaryngol 1985; 111:643–9.

5. Dipak Ranjan Nayak,Ramaswamy Balakrishnan, Deepak Murty K and Produl Hazarika. Endoscopic septoturbinoplasty: our update series Indian Journal of Otolaryngology and Head and Neck Surgery, 2002:54(1):20–22.

6. Nayak DR, Balakrishnan R and Murthy KD. An endoscopic approach to deviated nasal septum—a preliminary study. Journal of Laryngology and Otology 1998:112; 934–939.

7. Nayak DR, Satish R, Shah Parul, Poojary K and Balakrishnan R. Endoscopic Dacryocystorhinostomy and retrograde nasolacrimal duct dilatation with canulation—our experience. Indian Journal of Otolaryngology and Head and Neck Surgery 1999–2000: 52(1): 23–7, ISSN 0019–5421.

8. Rice DN. Endoscopic dacryocystorhinostomy: a cadaveric study. 1998; Ann of rhinol, 2, 127–8.

9. Nayak DR, Balakrishna R and Murthy KD. Endoscopic Physiologic Approach to Allergy associated chronic rhinosinusitis—a preliminary study , ENT Journal 2001: 80(6):392–403.

10. Dipak Ranjan Nayak, Suresh Pillai, Balakrishnan R, et al. Traditional Versus Transnasal Endoscopic Adenoidectomy—a comparative study. Indian Journal of Otolaryngology and Head and Neck Surgery 2005: Special Issue 1: 383–7.

11. DR Nayak, S Pillai and L Rao. Rhinofacial Zygomycosis caused by conidiobolus coronatus. Indian Journal of Otolaryngology and Head and Neck Surgery 2004:56(3):225–7.

12. Deepak Ranjan Nayak, Balkrishnan R and KD Murty. Turbinoplasty–letters to the Editor No. 2(reply) Ear, Nose and Throat Journal 2000.

13. "Paecilomyces infection of the paranasal sinuses in a child—a case report" Nayak DR. International Journal of Pediatric Otolaryngology, 2000:52: 183–187.

14. Nayak DR, Balakrishnan R and Adolph. Endoscopic adenoidectomy in Scheie's syndrome (MPS IS). International Journal of Pediatric Otolaryngology 1998: 44; 177–81.

15. Murthy PS, Sahota JS and Nayak DR, Balakrishnan R, Hazarika P. Foreign Body in the ethmoid sinus. International Journal of Oral and Maxillofacial Surgery 1994:23; 74–5.

16. Friedman WH, Katsantonis GP. The role of standard technique in modern sinus surgery. *OtolaryngolClin North Am.* 1989; 22:759–77.

17. Nayak DR and Balakrishnan R. Exclusive Endoscopic/Endoscopic-Assisted Minimally Invasive Surgery for Sinonasal Neoplasm—Our Experience; J Neurol Surg; B 2012; 73–A015.

# 6

# Preoperative Imaging Studies of the Nose and PNS

*Dr R Balakrishna*

Inflammatory disease of the paranasal sinuses is a common but serious health problem that can be associated with life threatening complications at times. Endoscopic sinus surgery has become a popular and effective surgical technique for treating patients with refractory inflammatory sinus disease.

The knowledge of the dominant role of the ethmoid sinus and the micro-architectural pathway between the sinuses and the nasal cavity in the pathogenesis, has paved the way for effective management of various nasal and paranasal sinus pathology. The success of functional endoscopic sinus surgery is facilitated by a clear understanding and therefore an accurate display of the anatomy of the nasal cavity and of the paranasal sinuses and their drainage pathways (especially the osteomeatal unit) in a plane correlating to the surgical orientation (Melhem, 1996).

Functional endoscopic sinus surgery even though is effective and popular is not always safe. This is because of the proximity of the spheno-ethmoid complex to the various vital structures, making them vulnerable to injury. Thus proper preoperative evaluation of the cases is mandatory. The CT scan imaging and diagnostic nasal endoscopy give comple-mentary information and remain the mainstay of preoperative evaluation of such cases. Direct coronal computed tomography (CT) of sinonasal anatomy displayed by using inter-mediate window and level settings (window 511700 Hounsfield units [HU], level 52300 HU) has been established as the imaging technique of choice for examining patients

before functional endoscopic sinus surgery because of its simulation of the surgical orientation, adequate depiction of bony and soft-tissue landmarks, and ability to show disease processes (Kennedy *et al.* 1985, Zenreich *et al.* 1987).

Melhem *et al.* (1996) proposed an optimal scanning protocol for the examination of the paranasal sinuses using a direct coronal plane with a scanning angle not exceeding 108 from the plane perpendicular to the hard palate, 3 mm thick contiguous sections, exposure factors of kV(p) 5–120, mA 5–80, detail reconstruction algorithm, and intermediate window settings (window 5–11700 HU, level 5–2300 HU). This protocol will provide excellent anatomic definition and orientation of the paranasal sinuses while significantly decreasing the radiation dose equivalent to patients.

## Role of Plain Radiographs

Clinically maxillary and frontal sinusitis is seen more frequently than the ethmoid sinus disease. Also the standard plain radiographs of the paranasal sinuses readily demonstrate the maxillary and frontal disease but not the ethmoidal disease, even though it is crucial in the pathogenesis.

## Advantages of Plain Radiographs

a. Quick, non-invasive and relatively inex-pensive.
b. It is possible to evaluate the maxillary, frontal, sphenoid sinuses and to some

53

extent the posterior ethmoid and lower third of nasal cavity.

c. Along with the clinical data, it helps to distinguish three types of nasosinus inflammatory disease, viz. rhinitis, rhino-sinusitis and polyposis.

d. Helps in optimal medical and conservative treatment including antral lavage and thus in attaining a more quiescent state of disease necessary for CT imaging.

### Disadvantages of Plain Radiographs

1. Gives no information regarding the ethmoid sinus-osteomeatal complex disease.

2. Gives no information regarding the position and status of the various vital structures related to the sphenoethmoids like the orbit, anterior cranial fossa, optic nerve and the internal carotid artery.

3. Extent of disease within the sphenoethmoids is not well delineated (Fig. 6.1).

### Role of CT Imaging

In contrast to the plain radiographs the CT imaging gives information regarding all the above mentioned under the disadvantages of plain radiographs.

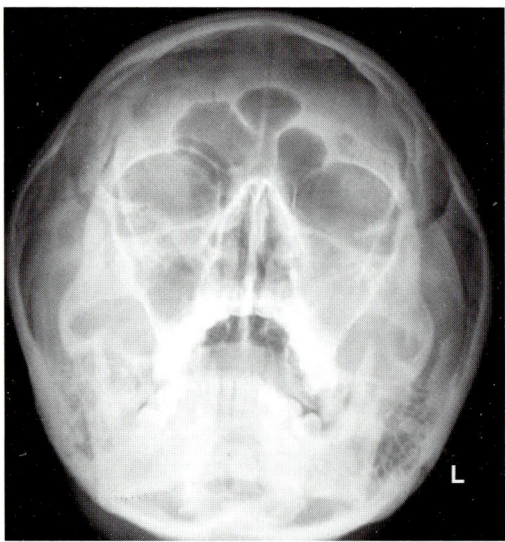

**Fig. 6.1:** Plain radiograph of paranasal sinuses showing haziness of both maxillary antrum

### Advantages of CT Imaging

1. CT imaging provides a precise knowledge of various sinus involved and thus allows the surgeon to tailor his surgery to the affected sinuses. When posterior ethmoids and sphenoids are found to be normal, there is no need to exenterate these, thus reducing the possibility of potential complications (Figs 6.2a and b).

2. CT scan provides information regarding the various anatomical and pathological variations in the osteomeatal complex. Apart from detecting the variations in the uncinate process, middle turbinate and bulla ethmoidalis, the CT scans also help in detecting the overpneumatized agger cells, frontal cells and Haller cells (Figs 6.2c and 6.4a,b). Haller and the Onodi cells which are not detectable otherwise. The Haller cells are the infraorbital ethmoid cells which being in close relation to the maxillary sinus ostium could narrow the infundibulum (Figs 6.2a to c and 6.5).

3. Most crucial role of CT imaging is to provide the surgeon, information regarding the position and status of the vital structures in relation to the sphenoethmoids. The dehiscence in the papery thin lamina papyracea (Fig. 6.4) either developmental or due to previous surgery is easily picked up by the coronal CT scans. Low position of Fovea ethmoidalis or cribriform plate is a potentially dangerous anatomical variation. A possible CSF leak can be averted by detection of this. Fovea ethmoidalis could also be dehiscent, and when so, is usually in its descending medial part. The position of anterior ethmoidal artery is an important landmark as it is considered high risk area in endoscopic sinus surgery (Fig. 6.4).

An overpneumatization of the posterior ethmoids and/or the sphenoid increases the vulnerability of the optic nerve and the internal carotid artery, as they bulge into the sinuses in the lateral walls. In rare instances the thin bone separating the internal carotid artery from the posterior ethmoid and sphenoid may be dehiscent. Overpneumatized sphenoid may give rise to various

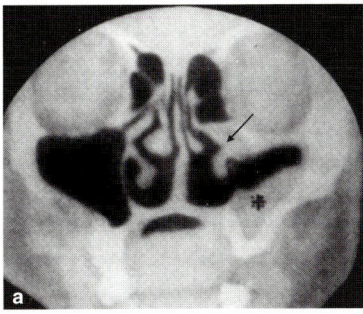
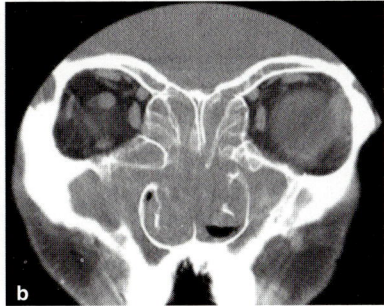
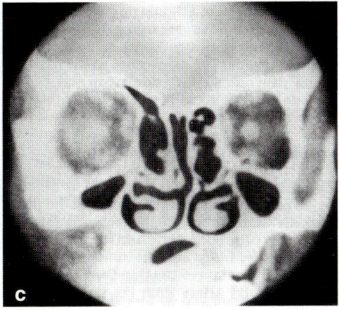

**Fig. 6.2: a.** CT imaging showing right maxillary disease (∗) in spite of a patent intranasal antrostomy infundibular disease and obstruction due to overpneumatized bulla and medially turned uncinate process are also seen (black arrow), **b.** CT picture in ethmoidal polyposis, **c.** CT scan showing overpneumatized bulla and medially bent uncinate process

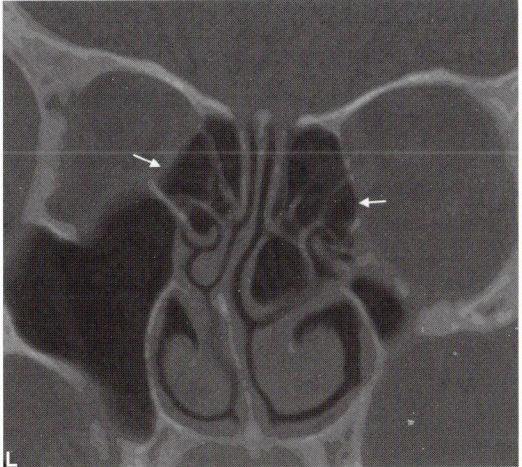

**Fig. 6.3:** CT scan showing paradoxically turned middle turbinate (right) and concha bullosa (left) and also note dehiscence fovea ethmoidalis and lamina papyracea (white arrows)

recesses like the anterior clinoid recess, pterygoid recess. Recess into the nasal septum or even into the greater wing of sphenoid. More the pneumatization, more is the chance for a complication (Fig. 6.5b). Identification of an asymmetric intersphenoid septum is important because the posterior extension of this partition usually marks the location of the internal carotid artery canal. Acute infection within the sphenoid can extend to the neighboring vital structure (Figs 6.5a, b and 6.6).

Marked lateral deviation or even fusion of uncinate process to the medial orbital wall may endanger the orbit while the uncinectomy is being performed.

The Onodi cells are the most posterior ethmoid cells that extend posterolaterally,

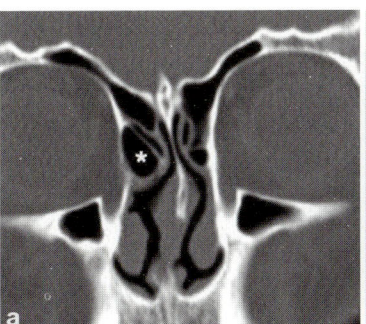
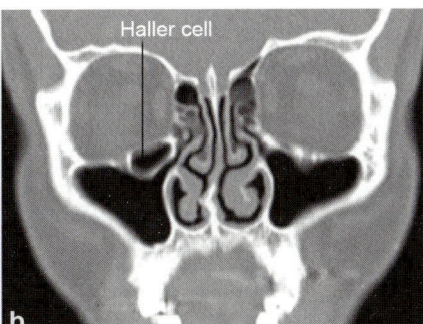
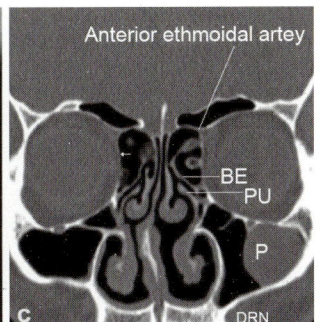

**Fig. 6.4: a.** CT scan showing overpneumatized agger cells, **b.** CT scan showing Haller cells, **c.** CT scan showing a dehiscent lamina papyracea associated with the right osteomeatal complex disease and bilateral antral polyp

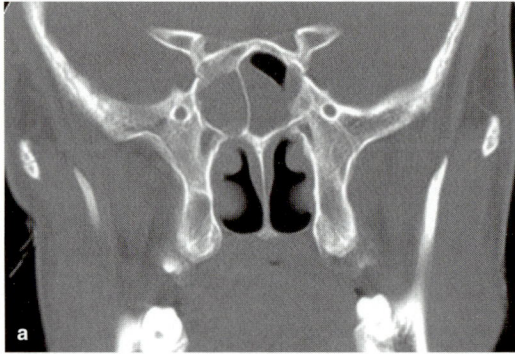

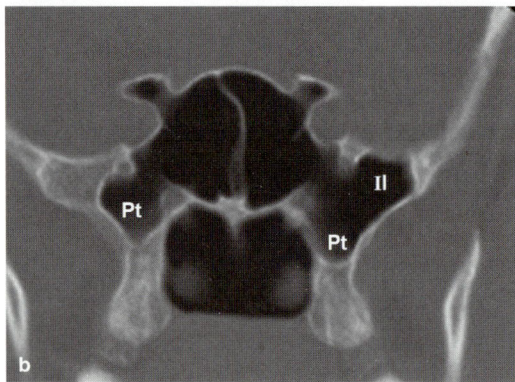

**Fig. 6.5: a.** CT scan showing sphenoidal sinusitis with fluid level on left side, **b.** CT scan showing bilateral pterygoid recesses (Pt), with an inferolateral recess on it (II) extending into the floor of the left middle cranial fossa in continuity with the pterygoid recess

and surround the optic canal and optic nerve. These cells may extend more posteriorly and protrude into the sphenoid sinuses as well as migrate to reach the anterior wall of the sella (para-sphenoidal posterior ethmoid) (Fig. 6.8).

4. CT scan imaging is a rapid, non-invasive and convenient investigation.
5. Helps in documentation and education.

### Disadvantages of CT Imaging

1. Relatively expensive investigation.
2. Radiation dose to the sensitive lens and cornea is particularly high when axial cuts are taken nearly 185 times the dose to the sensitive cornea and lens than that recorded for plain radiographs. This can be reduced by careful positioning of the patient in the scanner and by favouring more coronal cuts.
3. Artefacts due to extensive dental fillings. Here again coronal sections are better than axial sections.

### Coronal Versus Axial Cuts

Coronal CT scans are preferred as it displays structures in a plane closest to the endoscopist. Also the anatomical and pathological variations in the OMC are well delineated in the coronal cuts. The relation of cribriform plate,

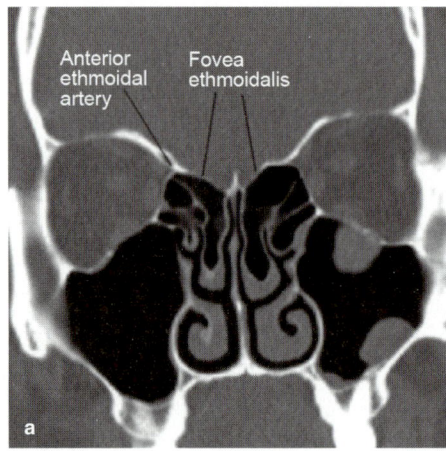

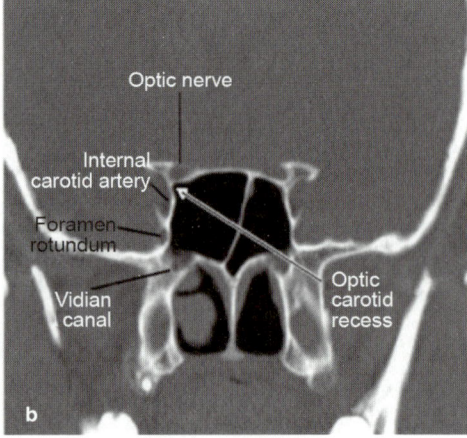

**Fig. 6.6: a.** CT scan showing dehiscence fovea ethmoidalis with polyps in left maxillary sinus. Also note the entry of anterior ethmoidal artery, **b.** CT scan showing the recess between the bulge of the optic nerve and carotid artery within the sphenoid sinus. Also note foramen rotundum and the vidian canal

fovea ethmoidalis, the lamina papyracea, the optic bulge and ICA bulge are better appreciated in coronal cuts.

The coronal CT scan of the paranasal sinuses is performed with the patient in the prone position with the head hyper-extended, 3 mm of thin coronal section are obtained from the frontal sinus to sphenoid sinus. The CT scan images should be photographed on bone (average 2000 H windows) setting as well as soft tissue (average 250 H windows) settings.

The coronal CT allows to study the level of the cribriform plate and the olfactory fossa as described by Kero's. This includes—(a) Kero's Type-1: olfactory fossa 1–3 mm deep, Type-2: olfactory fossa 4–7 mm deep, Type-3: olfactory fossa 8–16 mm deep (Fig. 6.6c).

The anterior and posterior walls of frontal sinus, the anatomical relationship between the posterior ethmoid and sphenoid sinuses and relationship of optic nerve to posterior ethmoid/sphenoid and pterygopalatine fossa are best evaluated in the axial planes. The axial cuts also help in delineating well the frontal sinus drainage pathway (frontal recess) and sphenoethmoidal recess.

Newer MDCT scanner allows taking 64 slices with each scanner rotation permitting high resolution multiplanner reformatted images. Use of this multiplanner reformation

(sagittal and coronal) has been shown to improve preoperative understanding of the frontal recess. Review of sagittal images significantly helps in identifying and measure the frontal recess and assessing the obstructing anterior ethmoid (Kew *et al.* 2002). Three-dimensional, reformatted images of frontonasal anatomy enable improved understanding of the frontal sinus drainage pathway, anatomy and of the spatial relationships between ethmoid air cells in this region (Fig. 6.7). Such images may provide a useful adjunct to surgical planning.

Axial cuts may be taken along with coronal and sagittal reconstruction. CT evidence of

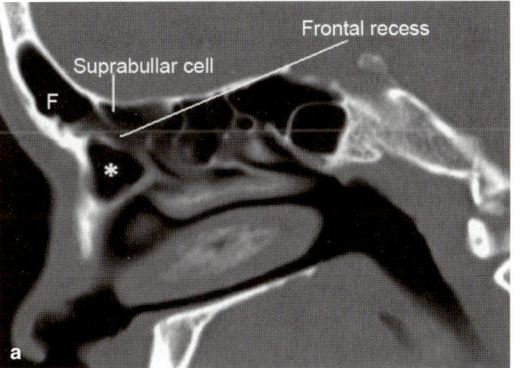

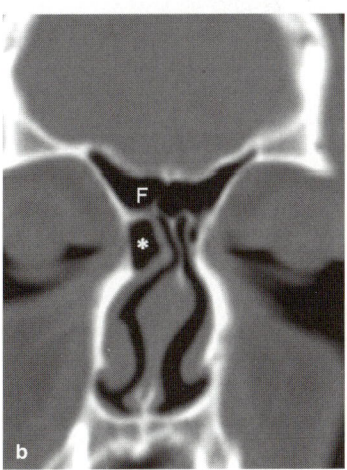

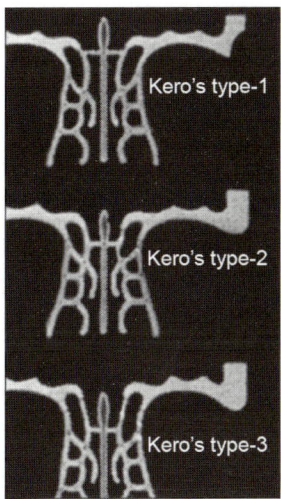

**Fig. 6.6c:** Level of cribriform plate

**Fig. 6.7: a.** Sagittal reconstruction, **b.** Coronal section Osteomeatal complex CT of paranasal sinus with prominent agger nasi cell (∗). Also note frontal recess and suprabullar cell shown in fig(a) marked with white line and frontal sinus (F)

hyperattenuation within spho-enethmoid should raise suspicion of allergic fungal sinusitis. MRI helps in soft tissue deleniation especially in orbital/intracranial complications of sinusitis. It also readily differentiates mucus from the mucosal disease.

## The Cost Effectiveness of CT Imaging

Keeping in mind the possibility of major complication that could result following an endoscopic sinus surgery, like blindness, orbital hematoma, CSF rhinorrhea, major ICA/Cavernous bleeding, etc. CT scan is definitely a cost effective investigation.

The cost effectiveness of CT scan imaging can be increased by

a. Lowering the cost (by reducing the number of films).

b. Increasing the effectiveness.

Many efforts are made to achieve this by taking lesser but strategically placed cuts (The mini series technique of White *et al.* 1990 and the limited scanning technique White *et al* 1991). Selective coronal and axial cuts are taken in the above technique.

## Pre-requisite before CT Imaging

As the objective of the CT imaging is to detect the subtle changes in the OMC causing the chronic sinusitis, and not the result of it, the CT scan should be taken only after proper medical and conservative procedures like antral wash, etc. to treat the disease in the major sinuses. The CT scan should be taken in a more quiescent state of the disease. A short course of steroid is helpful.

## Technique (Zenreich *et al.* 1987) Table 6.1

- Position: Prone with hyperextended head for coronal sections.
- CT specifications as per table.
- Window width around 2000 preferred and window centered to 200.
- When patient is unable to resume hyperextended head position, axial cuts are taken and coronal indirect reconstructions can be made.
- Initially, a sagittal scout section is taken and the coronal cuts are strategically

placed between the frontal and sphenoid sinuses. About 12 coronal cuts are usually sufficient. Infraorbital meatal line is drawn and cuts taken in the perpendicular or parallel to it for coronal and axial cuts respectively.

## Reporting of CT Films

A proforma followed by our institute for recording the findings is given below.

## Proforma

1. *Extent of the disease (T: Mucosal thickening, O: Complete opacity, C: Cloudiness)*
   a. Max. sinus (Polyp/fluid level)
   b. Frontal sinus
   c. Anterior ethmoids
   d. Middle ethmoid
   e. Posterior ethmoids
   f. Sphenoid
   g. Infundibulum
      (Patent = N; Partial occlusion = +; Total occlusion = + +)
   h. Middle meatus (N/Narrow)
   i. Polyps (+/−)
   j. Frontal recess (status of agger nasi and frontal cell/cells)
   k. Sphenoethmoidal recess
   l. Sinus lateralis
   m. Focal or diffuse area of attenuation.
   n. Other changes (bone/mucocele, etc.).

2. *Anatomical and pathological variations*
   a. Agger nasi cells
   b. Haller cells
   c. Overpneumatized bulla
   d. Uncinate process—medially turned, laterally turned, up bulla.
   e. Middle turbinate—concha bullosa, bulky MT, paradoxically turned MT
   f. Onodi cells
   g. Septal deviation
   h. Post-traumatic structural variations (including surgical, if any).
   i. Others

3. *Danger points*
   a. Cribriform plate

| Imaging Parameter | Imaging Plane | |
|---|---|---|
| | **Coronal** | **Axial** |
| Patient position | Prone | Supine |
| Gantry angulations | Perpendicular to IOML | IOML |
| Extent of study | From anterior frontal sinus to posterior sphenoid sinus | From hard palate through frontal sinus |
| Section thickness (mm) | 4 | 4 |
| Table incrementation (mm) | 3 | 3 |
| kVp | 125 | 125 |
| mAs | 450 | 450 |
| Scan time (sec) | 5 | 5 |

**Table 6.1:** Technique for CT of paranasal sinuses

b. Fovea ethmoidalis
c. Lamina papyracea (can be involved due to extensive ethmoidal polyposis) (Fig. 6.2b)
d. Relation of ICA/optic nerve to posterior ethmoids and sphenoids.
e. Lacrimal bone/duct.

## Friedman's CT Staging of Chronic Hyperplastic Rhinosinusitis

*Stage I :* Single focus disease.
*Stage II:* Multifocal disease responsive to conservative therapy.
*Stage III:* Diffuse disease partially responsive to medication.

*Stage IV:* Diffuse disease with bony changes and poorly responding to conservative therapy.

The staging is said to be useful in outlining operative strategies and a reliable prognostic indicator of the disease process. To sum-marize, CT imaging is a useful and essential tool to the rhinologist for performing endo-scopic sinus surgery. It allows the surgeon to tailor his surgery to the affected sinuses, treat adequately and effectively the casual anato-mical variation and pathological changes in the OMC and at the same time alarms the surgeon of the possibility of an avertable complication due to FESS, thus making the surgery both effective as well as safe and thus an efficient one.

## REFERENCES AND FURTHER READING

1. Zenreich et al. Paranasal sinuses-CT imaging requirements for endoscopic surgery. Radiology 163, 1987; pp. 769–75.

2. Kennedy et al. FESS - Part I - Theory and diagnostic evaluation. Arch Otolaryngol Vol 111 Sept. 1985, 576–82.

3. Llyod et al. CT of paranasal sinuses and FESS. A critical analysis of 100 symptomatic patients. JLO, March 1991, Vol 105; pp 181–5.

4. Bolger et al. Paranasal sinus surgery—anatomic variations and mucosal abnormalities. CT analysis for endoscopic sinus surgery. Laryngoscope 101 Jan. 1991, pp 56–64.

5. Mafee MF. Preoperative imaging anatomy of nasal ethmoid complex for FESS. RCNA Vol. 31, No. 1, Jan. 1993; pp 1–20.

6. Paul S White. Limited CT scanning techniques of the PNS. JLO Jan. 1991 Vol. 105; pp 20–3.

7.  Dale H Rice: Basic surgical techniques and variations of endoscopic sinus surgery. OCNA Vol 2 No. 4 Aug. 1989, pp 713–726.

8.  Friedman CT staging of PNS in Chronic hyperplast rhinosinusitis. Laryngoscope 100 Nov. 1990, pp 1161–1165.

9.  Elias R. Melhem, Patrick J Oliverio, Mark L Benson, Optimal CT Evaluation for Functional Endoscopic Sinus Surgery; Am. J Neuroradiol 17:181–188, January 1996.

10. Kew J et al. Multiplanar reconstructed computed tomography images improves depiction and understanding of the anatomy of the frontal recess and frontal sinus, Am. J Rhinology, 2002, 16(2):119–23.

# 7

# Premedication and Preoperative Management

Proper preoperative counseling and adequate preparation of the patient prior to endoscopic sinus surgery is mandatory for a smooth and effective conduction of endoscopic sinus surgery. Serious complications usually result from impaired visibility due to excessive bleeding during surgery.

To avoid such complications, endoscopic sinus surgery can be performed either with local anesthesia with vasoconstrictors (Friedman 1996), or under general anesthesia supplemented with controlled hypotension (Heermann 1999). The preparation should be done in the following lines:

1. Adequate control of active infection by appropriate antibiotics, nasal deconge-stants (topical and systemic) and anti-histaminic.

2. More quiescent the state of the disease, less is the possibility of hemorrhage intra-operatively, thus allowing the endoscopic sinus surgery to be more effective.

3. In case of polyposis, oral steroids, like prednisolone 5 mg tid for a week prior to surgery, will help in either reducing the size of polyp or at times even causing disappearance of the polyp. With this, the intraoperative bleeding will be less and the surgeon can completely exenterate the ethmoids.

4. Preoperative evaluation should concen-trate towards finding out the other causes which could lead to intraoperative bleed-ing like hypertension, bleeding diatheses, history of concommitant aspirin or warfarin therapy, etc. ESS should be performed after tackling the above factors. The routine work-up of the patient should hence includes

   a. A complete blood picture like Hb, PCV, total and differential count, etc.
   b. Estimation of bleeding, clotting and prothrombin times and
   c. Urine analysis for albumin and sugar.

5. A Xylocaine sensitivity test is advocated prior to surgery.

Patient is ideally hospitalised a day prior to surgery for the preparation and investi-gations. Oral Diazepam 5–10 mg is given at night previous day to the surgery and also in the morning next day about 4 hrs before surgery. This helps in reducing anxiety and thus preventing a possible rise in blood pressure. The patient is advised to stay Nil per oral overnight prior to surgery.

## Premedication for FESS under Local Anesthesia

The following premedication is given 45 minutes prior to surgery

1. Inj. Pethidine 1–1.5 mg/kg body weight (approximately 75–100 mg in an average adult patient).

2. Inj. Phenergan 25 mg.

3. Inj. Atropine 0.6 mg.

These are given together deep intra-muscular about 45 minutes before the surgery. Pethidine is a very potent narcotic analgesic, the action of which is synergised by phener-gan. Phenergan in addition combats the side effect of nausea and vomiting due to pethidine. Increased dose of pethidine is preferred rather than use of largactil, a tranquilliser, as it gives better analgesia and patient will have fewer hallucinations.

Atropine helps in reducing the nasal secretions, thus giving a dry operative field. Also being a vagolytic, it is cardio protective. Oral opioids are commonly prescribed after sinus surgery but are associated with adverse effects, including gastrointestinal and neurologic symptoms. Nonopioid analgesics have been suggested to offer similar pain control efficacy with fewer adverse effects.

## Premedication for FESS under GA

Clonidine, a potent suppressor of sympatho-adrenal activity, has been given orally before operation to augment the hypotensive action of isoflurane. The antihypertensive drug, clonidine, is a centrally acting alpha 2 agonist, useful as a premedication because of its sedative and analgesic properties and provides a clear field, it also reduces bleeding effectively during intraoperative period during endoscopic sinus surgery (Jabalameli *et al*. 2005).

## Ontable Preparation

Cottonoid strips are made by cutting the soft roll rayon pads available commercially, into strips of 3 × 1.5 cm and a black cotton or silk thread about 1 foot long is stitched to one end of the strip as in Fig. 7.1. Such strips are made into a bundle and are sterilized by autoclaving. Such cottonoids are dipped in a solution containing 10 ml of 4% xylocaine and 1 ml of 1:1000 adrenaline thus making the dilution of adrenaline into 1:10,000. The strips are squeezed and 4–5 such strips are used per nasal for preoperative packing, after sparying the nasal cavity with 4% xylocaine spray. The packs are placed by direct visualization using nasal endoscope. Sites of placement are as follows:

1. Posteriorly in the middle meatus and as close to the sphenopalatine foramen as possible
2. Between the lateral wall and middle turbinate anteriorly

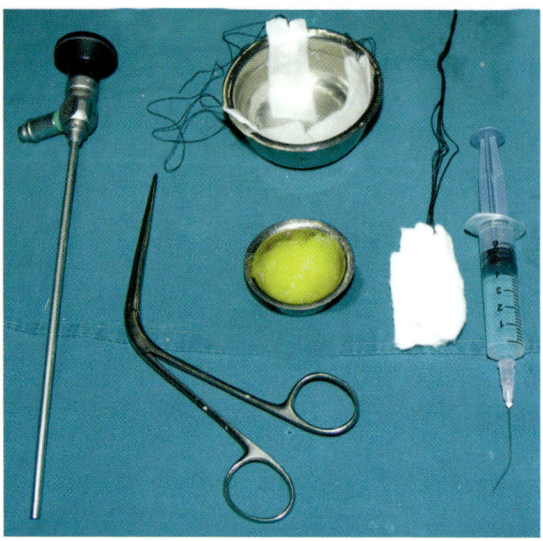

**Fig. 7.1:** 10 ml 4% xylocaine with 1:1000 adrenaline solution cottonoids strip nasal endoscope and nasal dressing forceps required for placement of strips in the middle meatus and nasal cavity, syringe for 2% xylocaine with in 1:100000 adrenaline for infiltration

3. Between the middle turbinate and septum
4. Between the inferior turbinate and the septum (1 or 2 strips).

This gives good surface anesthesia as well as decongests the turbinates, increasing the exposure of the operative field. Thus handling of the nasal endoscope and other instruments is made easy and less painful.

Antifog solution like savlon or sterile dilute soap water solution is used to prevent fogging of the tip of nasal endoscope.

**Intraoperative treatment:** Saline irrigations were found to significantly reduce the amount of *S. pneumoniae* found within the maxillary sinus mucosa. No difference was found for *H. influenzae* in bacterial load reduction which was noted between the pressurized saline flushes and manual saline rinse methods (Kristine *et al*. 2011).

Data analysis have shown significant improvement in early postoperative healing in sinonasal cavities receiving triamcinolone-impregnated absorbable nasal packing following ESS and is also associated with significantly improved healing up to 6 months postoperatively (Cote and Wright *et al.* 2010). The author (DRN) in his personal experience also found significant improve- ment in healing while using hydrocortisone and povidone iodine impregnated absorbable nasal packing with no systemic side effects.

## REFERENCES AND FURTHER READING

1. Jabalameli *et al.* Oral Clonidine Premedication Decreases Intraoperative Bleeding in Patients Undergoing Endoscopic Sinus Surgery; Journal of Research in Medical Sciences 2005; 1: 25–30.

2. Friedman M, Venkatesan TK, Lang D, Caldarelli DD. Bupivacaine for postoperative analgesia following endoscopic sinus surgery. Laryngoscope, 1996; 106(11):1382–5.

3. Heermann J, Neues D. Intranasal microsurgery of all paranasal sinuses, the septum and the lacrimal sac with hypotensive anesthesia, Ann oral rhinol laryngol, 1999; 95: 631–8.

4. Christopher A. *et al.* Rofecoxib versus Hydrocodone/Acetaminophen for Postoperative Analgesia in Functional Endoscopic Sinus Surgery; Laryngoscope. 116(4):602–606, April 2006.

5. Kristine *et al.* Effect of intraoperative saline irrigation on bacterial load within the maxillary sinus; International Forum of allergy and rhinology, 2011; V-1(5): 351–355.

6. David WJ Cote and Erin D Wright: Triamcinolone-impregnated nasal dressing following endoscopic sinus surgery—A randomised double blind placebo control study; Laryngoscope, 2010; (120)1269–73.

# 8

# Endoscopic Sinus Surgery—Instruments, Disinfection and Sterilization

## Instrumentation for Diagnostic Nasal Endoscopy and Endoscopic Sinus Surgery

1. 7210 A. Hopkins II Forward-Oblique Telescope 30°, diameter 4 mm, length 18 cm. Used for diagnostic nasal endoscopy and during surgery in the frontal recess and maxillary sinus ostium (Fig. 8.1).

2. 7210 AA. Hopkins II Straightforward Telescope 0°. Diameter 4 mm, length 18 cm. Used for endoscopic sinus surgery (Fig. 8.2).

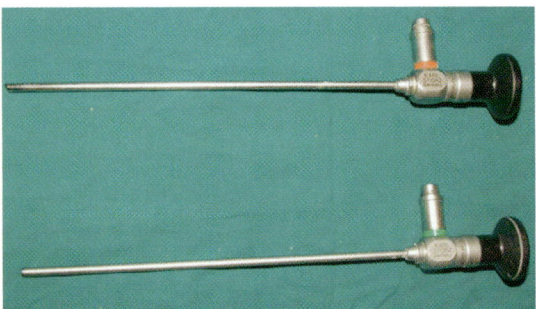

**Fig. 8.1:** Hopkins 0° straightforward and 30° oblique telescope

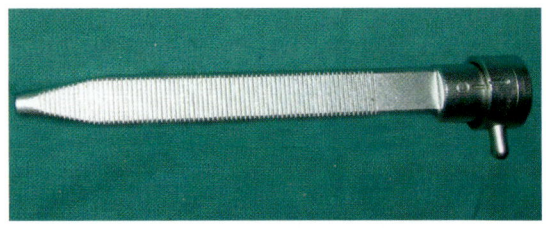

**Fig. 8.2:** Stammberger telescope handle

3. 723770 Stammberger telescope handle for use with straightforward telescope degree.

4. 27018 A. Hopkins Straightforward Telescope 0°, diameter 2.7 mm, length 18 cm. Used for endoscopic sinus surgery in pediatric age group patients.

5. 27018 B. Hopkins Forward-Oblique Telescope 30°, diameter 2.7 mm, length 18 cm. Used for diagnostic nasal endoscopy in pediatric age group patients.

6. 722830. Suction tube, inch finger cut-off, working length 14 cm, size 3 mm.

7. 586230. Suction tube, short curved, 15 cm, size 3 mm.

8. 456001 B. Rhinoforce Blakesly nasal forceps, straight, 19 cm. working length 10 cm, size 1.

9. 457001 B. Rhinoforce Strumpel-Voss nasal forceps, 45° upturned, working length 10 cm, size 1.

10. 455000 B. Rhinoforce Takahashi nasal forceps, straight, working length 10 cm.

11. 449201 Rhinoforce nasal scissor, working length 13 cm, straight.

12. 459011 Rhinoforce Stammberger antrum Puncture working length 10 cms, right side backward cutting.

13. 459012 Rhinoforce Stammberger antrum Puncture working length 10 cm, left side backward cutting.

14. 628001 Sickle knife, pointed, 19 cm.

15. 474000 Freer elevator, double ended, length 20 cm.

16. 723772 Stammberger telescope handle, round.
17. 20112001 Cold light Fountain Halogen 150.
18. 20112025. Spare reflector lamp 150 W, 15 V.
19. 495 NB. Fibreoptic light cable. Size 4.8 mm, length 180 cm.
20. 486030 V. EICKEN antrum cannula, 15 cm. long curved, OD 3 mm, Luer-lock. (Fig. 8.3).
21. 723005 A. Trocar and Cannula for sinuscopy, OD 5 mm. Length of cannula 8.5 cm, fenestrated beck (Fig. 8.4).
22. Stortz endoscopic video camera and cable system (Fig. 8.5).
23. Xomed micro-debridor system (Fig. 8.6a and b).
24. Colour monitor

### Set Up

1. Patient's table
2. Double level instrument table: upper level—cottonoids, lower level—light source.
3. Mayo stand for the instruments and kidney tray filled with saline.

4. Adjustable stool for the surgeon.
5. Floor should be carpeted or padded; in case an endoscope or instrument falls, it will not get spoilt.

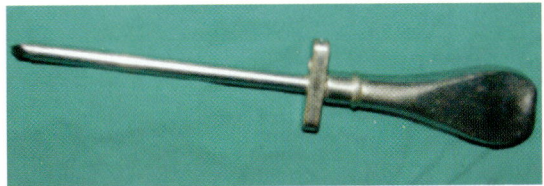

**Fig. 8.4:** Trocar and cannula for sinuscopy

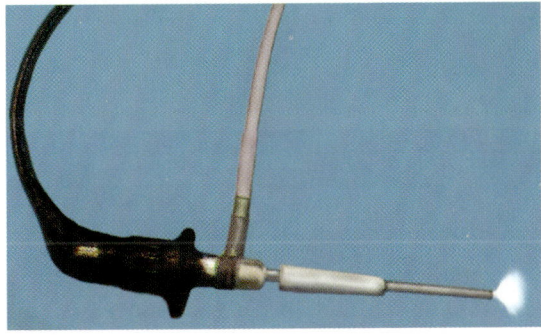

**Fig. 8.5:** Endoscope with camera attachment for video endoscopy, preferably HD camera

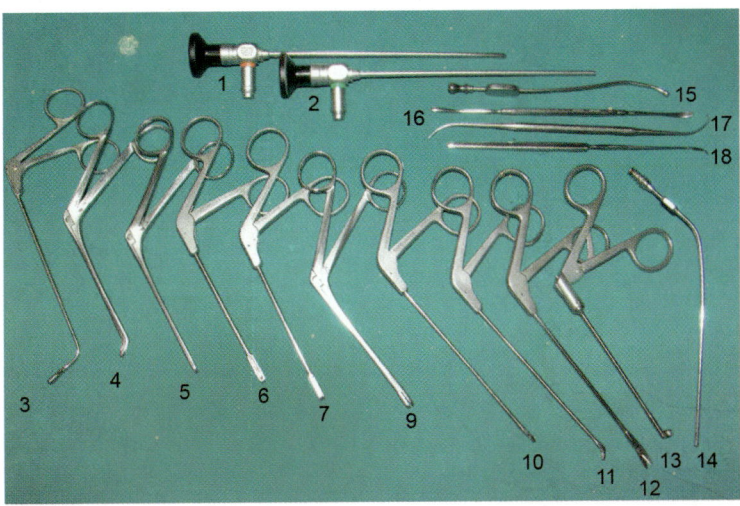

**Fig. 8.3:** 0 and 30 degree endoscope (1 and 2), 90 degree upturned Stammberger (Giraffe) forceps (3), Blakesley 45 and 0 degree forceps (4 and 5), Stammberger antrum puncture back biting right and left (6 and 7), Takahashi nasal forceps (9), Heuwieser through cutting tissue sparing forceps (10 and 11), Rhinoforce nasal scissors (12), Stammberger antrum punch down and forward cutting (13), Frazier suction tube (14), Curved suction cannula for frontal sinus (15), Mucoperichondrial elevator (16), Kuhn-Bolger frontal ostium seeker (17), Sickle knife (18)

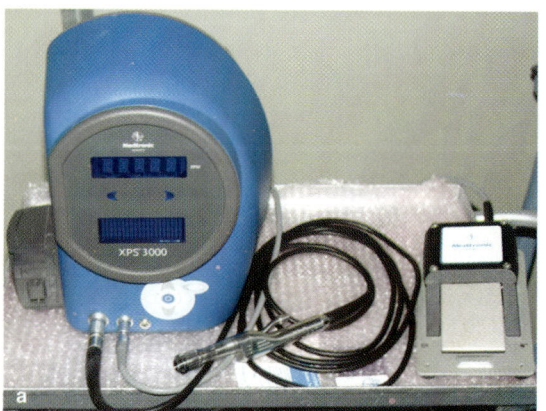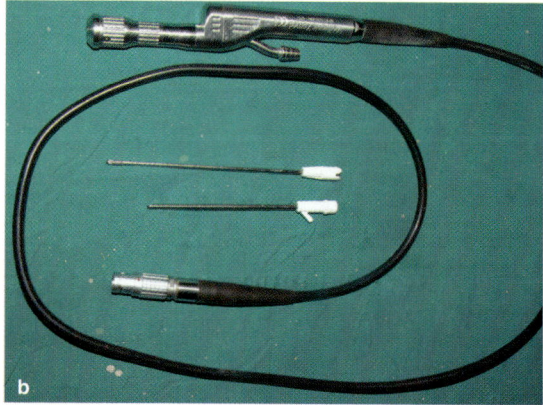

**Fig. 8.6: a.** Xomed microdebridor system for endoscopic sinus surgery, **b.** handpiece cable and blades

## Handling the Instruments

### Endoscope

It is held in the left hand like a pen. Extra grip can be attained by using the telescope handles (optional). The last 3 fingers of the left hand should rest on the patients face for proper stability. The tip of the endoscope is dipped in defogging solution, excess solution is wiped off, and then the endoscope is inserted into the nasal cavity. The surgeon should instruct the patient not to move his or her head and to inform him if the patient has pain or feels like sneezing. This is important as the patients movements can damage the delicate endoscopes and instruments.

### Powered Instrument System

The shaver (powered instrument) system offer different handpieces, knives, irrigation and modes (rotating or oscillating). Shaver is a combination of suction and cutting round knife working together. Knives of different shapes are put into handpiece. Shaver surgery is precise in soft tissue resection, so the most advantages to power the system is in rhino-surgery, polypectomy with extension to pansinus surgery (Dalke *et al.* 2006).

### Image Guidance Systems for Sinus Surgery

The electromagnetic-based Insta Trak® system and the optical-based Stealth-Station are commonly used for endoscopic sinus

surgery. Each system was noted to have limitations. The presence of metallic objects in the operative field interfered with functioning of the electromagnetic system, whereas the optical system required a clear line of sight to be maintained between the infrared camera and surgical handpiece. Both systems required specialized headsets to be worn by patients during surgery to monitor head position. The electromagnetic system also required these headsets to be worn during the preoperative computed tomography scan. Although both these two image guidance systems proved valuable for anatomic localization during sinus surgery, individual preferences can be based on distinct differences in their design and operation.

*Multiangle endoscope:* This endoscope developed by Acclarent Cyclops, has a shaft which rotates, giving an angle of view from 10 to 90 degrees. It is useful in minimally invasive sinus surgery and endoscopic skull base surgery avoiding repeated changing of scopes for angle vision (Fig. 8.7) besides, giving a costom desired angle of view.

### Disinfection of the Instruments

High-level disinfection provides a reasonably effective method of reducing bacterial and fungal contamination of fiberoptic nasal endoscope. Appropriate surveillance tech-nique should be used in each clinical setting

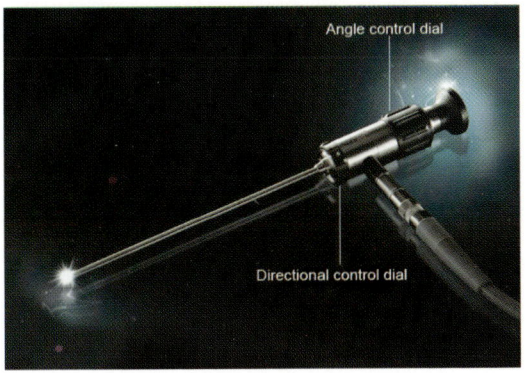

**Fig. 8.7:** Multiangle endoscope

before immersing in the activated solution. Cleanse and rinse the lumens of the suction tubes before filling with activated solution. Immerse completely for a minimum of 10 minutes. This destroys the vegetative organisms, pathogenic fungi and viruses. Remove the equipment from the activated solution and rinse thoroughly with sterile water prior to use.

Taking care of nasal endoscope is extremely important while performing the surgery. The tip of the nasal endoscope gets frequently soiled with blood. Unless cleaned regularly, the dried blood clot can decrease the longevity of the endoscope. The author prefers to clean the tip with normal saline, which is kept in a bowl with cotton being kept at the bottom. Recently endo-scrub 2 lens cleaning sheath has been introduced. This helps in continuing the surgery without withdrawing the scape for repeated cleaning. This system also prevents fogging, while performing endoscopy.

with flexible and rigid fiberoptic scopes to ensure adequate disinfection effectiveness.

This is done by using a 2% W/V solution of glutaraldehyde (Cidex®). Addition of the activator to this solution turns it bright green (activated solution). This can be used for a maximum period of 2 weeks, clean; rinse and rough dry the endoscopes and instruments

## REFERENCES AND FURTHER READING

1. Neil Bhattacharyya MD, and Lynne J Kepnes RNP[a] The effectiveness of immersion disinfection for flexible fiberoptic laryngoscopes Otolaryngology—Head and Neck Surgery, June 2004; Vol 130, Issue 6; 681–5.

2. Metson, Ralph MD; Laryngoscope. 108(8, Part 1): 1164–1170, A Comparison of Image Guidance Systems for Sinus Surgery August 1998.

3. Stortz the world of endoscopy, endoscopes and instruments for ENT 6th Edition.

4. Dalke et al. Rotation suction-knife (shaver) in otorhinolaryngological surgery. Otolaryngol Pol. 2006; 60(1):37–40.

# 9

# Messerklinger's Technique of Functional Endoscopic Sinus Surgery (FESS)

## Anesthesia

This can be done either under local anesthesia or general anesthesia, but local anesthesia is preferred. There is difference of opinion among otolaryngologists about the safest way to administer anesthesia during endoscopic sinus surgery. Most of the surgeons maintain that the risk of complications under general anesthesia is greater because of greater blood loss and poor visualization than with local anesthesia (Stankiewicz 1989), where vaso-constriction is better achieved. Moreover, the medial orbital wall, orbital periosteum and thinnest part of the skull base are sensitive to pain, facilitate careful monitoring in an awake patient. Thus major complications can be avoided and vision can be monitored. Local injection of a solution containing a vaso-constrictor is required in all cases regardless of the anesthesia chosen to minimize the bleeding. The surgical risk to the patient diminishes as the surgeons ability to visualize the field increases.

General anesthesia is given in children and in apprehensive patients. Topical anesthetic agent like 4% xylocaine with 1:100,000 adrenaline soaked in cottonoids are used for initial vasoconstriction. The cottonoids should be kept in the middle meatus, between the septum and the turbinates. This facilitates in increasing the area of access to the operative field and allows smooth passage of instruments through the nose without causing much discomfort to the patient. After 5 minutes, the medial infundibular wall, anterior end of

middle turbinate and ethmoidal bulla are injected with 2% xylocaine with (1:100,000) adrenaline under endoscope visualization (black dots shown in Fig. 9.2).

## Operative Technique

### Position of the Patient

The patient should be placed in the supine position with the head slightly elevated and turned towards the surgeon. The patient should be asked to breath through mouth, if the operation is performed using local anesthesia. A 0° nasal endoscope is used for most part of the surgery and this is the only endoscope to be used by the beginner as it gives a direct view. After getting well acquainted with the normal landmarks, one can start using angled endoscope (Fig. 9.1).

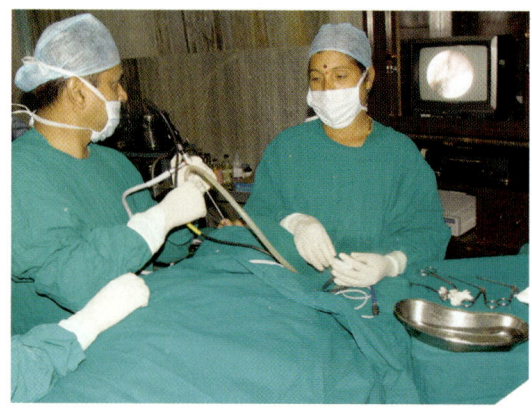

**Fig. 9.1:** Endoscopic assessment before starting FESS

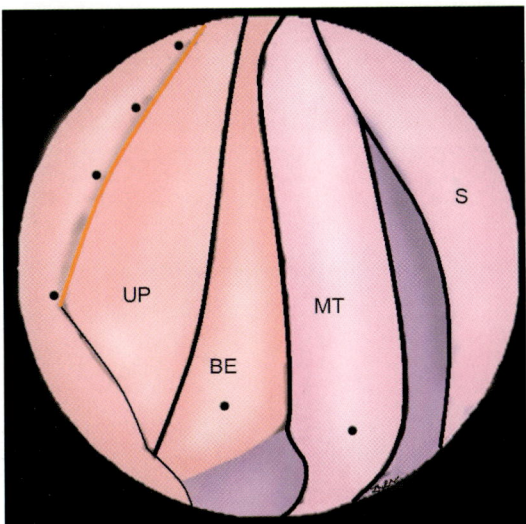

**Fig. 9.2:** Sites of local anesthetic infiltration on the uncinate process, bulla ethmoidalis and the middle turbinate

## Steps of Surgery

### Infundibulotomy (Uncinectomy)

After proper infiltration as in Fig. 9.2 incision is given circumferentially over the mucosa immediately anterior to the uncinate process using a sickle knife. The tip of the knife should be directed inferiorly and parallel to the lateral nasal wall to prevent injury to the lamina papyracea (Fig. 9.3).

After the incision, the uncinate process is subluxed medially with the help of a straight perichondrial elevator from its superior and inferior attachment (Figs 9.4 and 9.5a to d).

The superior insertion of the uncinate process is then carefully grasped with Blakesley-Weil forceps and is resected using endoscopic scissors and then separated from the lateral wall by a twisted motion of the forceps (Figs 9.6a and b).

Then the inferior portion is grasped and removed in a similar way. After infundibulum is opened, the surgeon can then determine if further procedure in the area of frontal recess or the ostium of the maxillary sinus is required.

## Anterior Ethmoidectomy and Middle Meatal Antrostomy

### Antrostomy

After infundibulotomy, the ostium of the maxillary sinus is frequently visible. Sometimes the posterior inferior remnant of the uncinate process prevents the visualization of the ostium and has to be removed. If the frontal sinus is involved, the way is open to

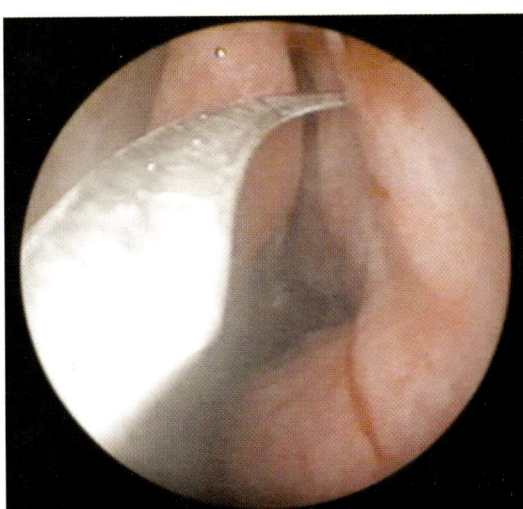

**Fig. 9.3:** Incision being given at the attachment of the uncinate process on the left side

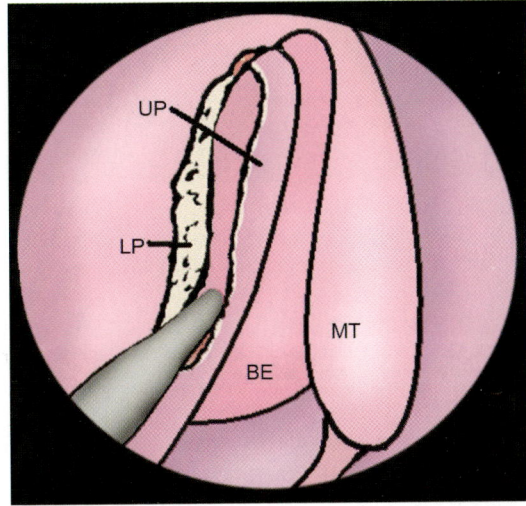

**Fig. 9.4:** The uncinate process being subluxed using an elevator on the right side

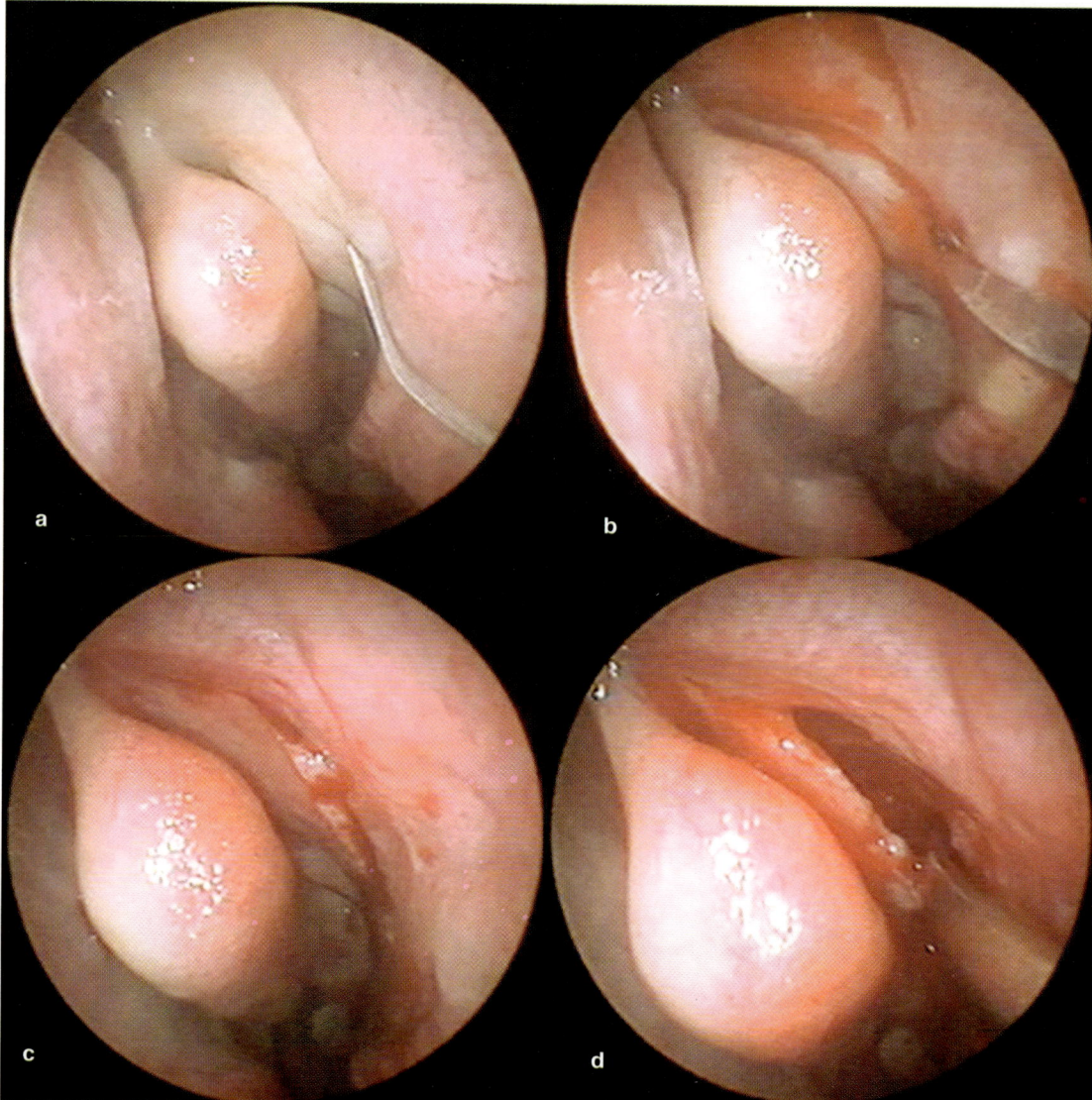

**Fig. 9.5:** Video endoscopic photograph showing the steps of infundibulotomy, **a.** infiltration along the uncinate process, **b.** incision is being given at the attachment site, **c.** showing the incised uncinate process before subluxation and **d.** subluxation of uncinate process is carried out by using a curved septal elevator (left)

the frontal recess. But in case the disease involves the ethmoidal bulla or posterior ethmoid and sphenoid, the disease has to be cleared from these areas before approaching the frontal recess to prevent troublesome bleeding that can complicate the surgical process unnecessarily.

The bulla ethmoidalis and anterior ethmoidal cells are removed by the Blakesly forceps. As the more superior cells are removed, care is taken to identify the ethmoidal roof. A beginner must use a zero degree scope for surgery of this region and should keep the upper attachment of the middle turbinate as the superior landmark, and should never go above that level to prevent injury to the dura. The bulla is opened by gently pushing on its anterior

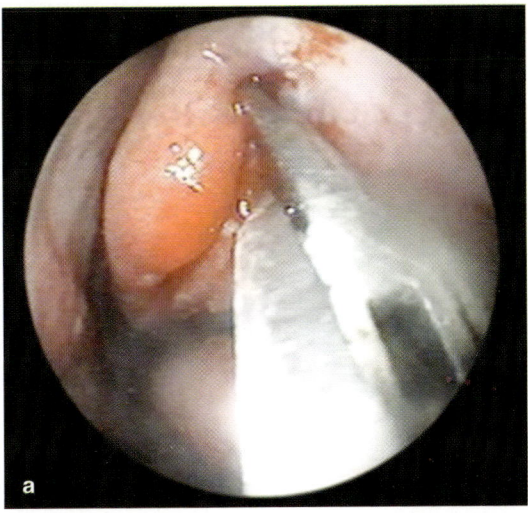

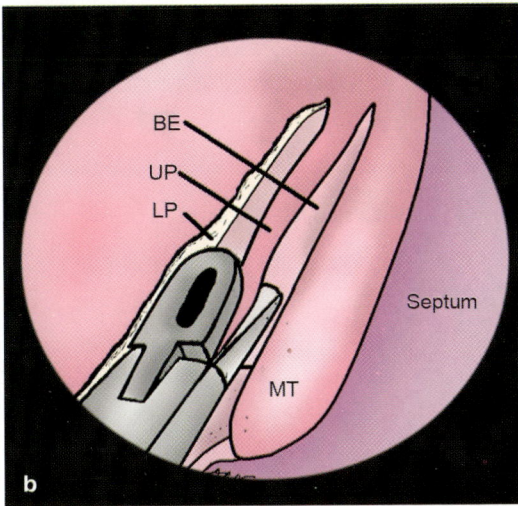

**Fig. 9.6: a.** Endoscopic picture showing subluxated uncinate process being divided, **b.** the uncinate process is grasped using Blakesly forceps before removal

surface in the medial direction with a delicate Blakesley-Weil forceps or a suction tip (Figs 9.7 and 9.8). After identifying the lumen the entire bulla can be resected step by step (Figs 9.9 and 9.10).

Above and anterior to bulla, there are 2–3 small ethmoidal cells and the sinus lateralis and can be removed if they are found to be diseased. While clearing the disease from the roof of the ethmoid, the position of the anterior ethmoidal artery should be kept in mind (Fig. 9.11).

The vessel passes across the ethmoid immediately below the anterior skull base in a partial or complete bony ridge attached to the ethmoidal roof as an useful landmark. If the anterior skull base is not identifiable, surgery in this area is deferred until ethmoidal

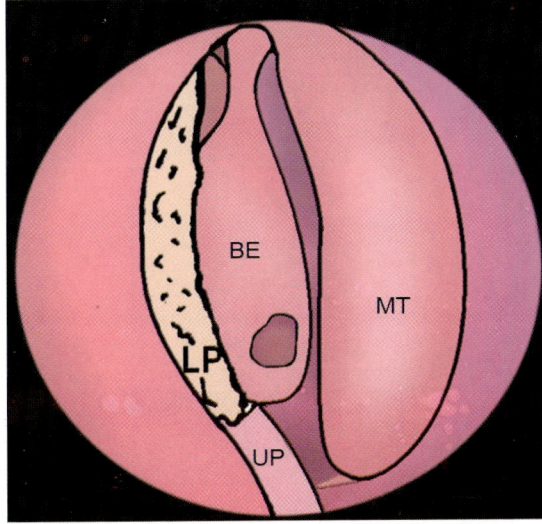

**Fig. 9.7:** Bulla ethmoidalis (left) being opened

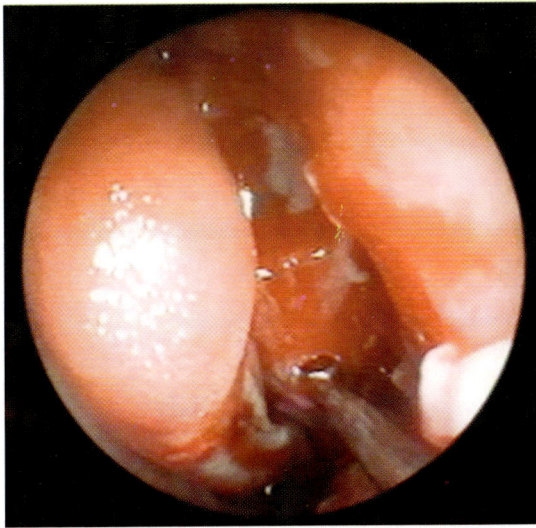

**Fig. 9.8:** Opened bulla ethmoidalis (right)

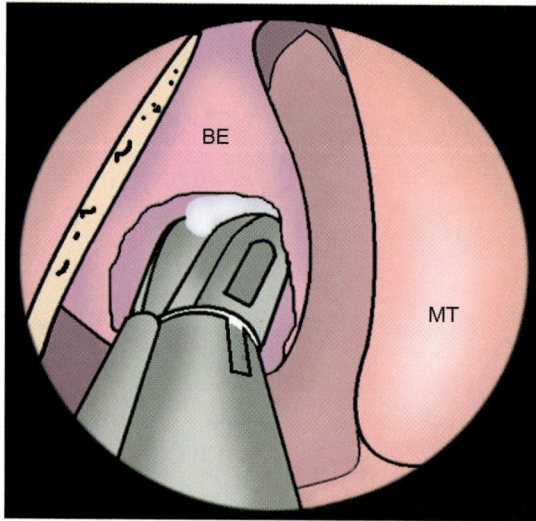

**Fig. 9.9:** Anterior ethmoidectomy being performed after opening of the bulla

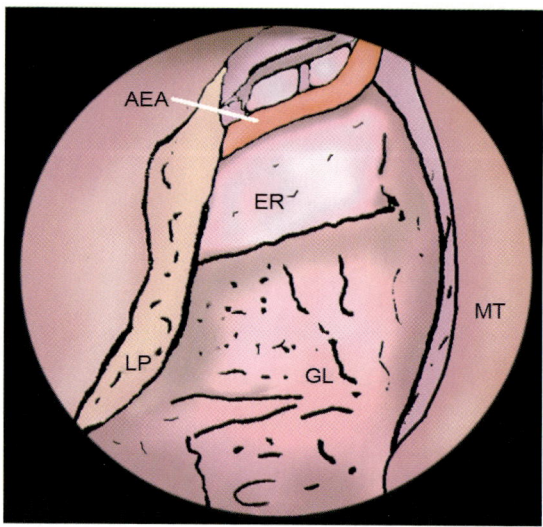

**Fig. 9.11:** Exposure of ground lamella (GL) after anterior ethmoidectomy (right)

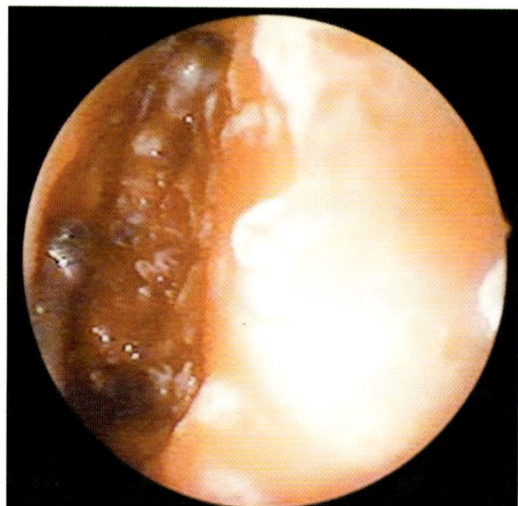

**Fig. 9.10:** Endoscopic picture showing bulla ethmoidalis is removed after complete infundibulotomy (left)

The maxillary sinus ostium is not enlarged routinely if the ostium is well patent. In case of stenosis, the ostium is enlarged towards the anterior fontanelle by using back biting forceps (Figs 9.13a and b), after identification of the ostium by palpation with a bent spoon.

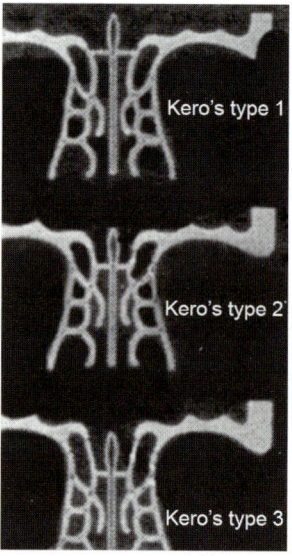

**Fig. 9.12:** Level of ethmoidal roof in relation to cribriform plate and middle turbinate

roof is identified within the poster ethmoid or sphenoid. CT imaging showing level of ethmoidal roof and cribriform plate is very important while dealing with the ethmoidal roof (Fig. 9.12).

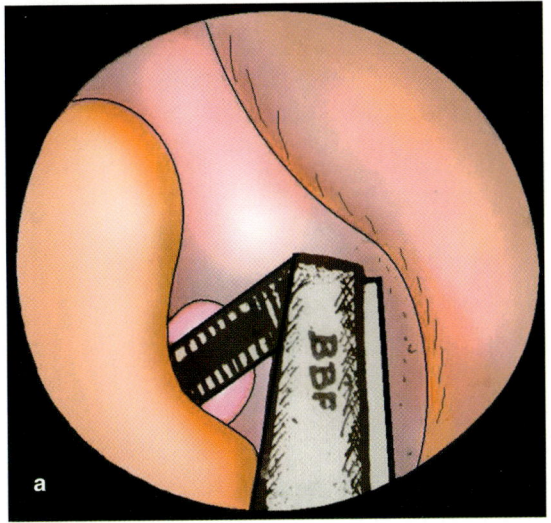

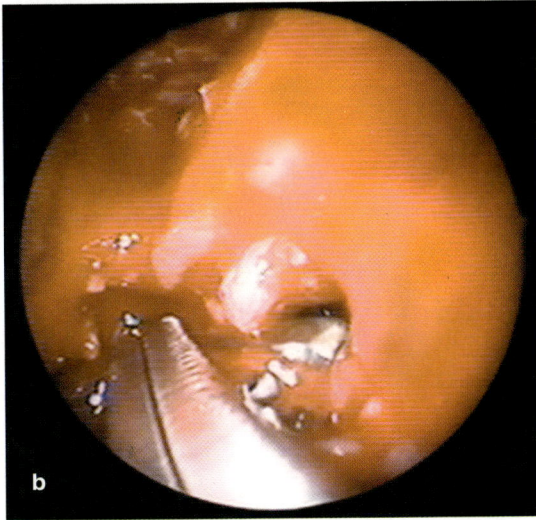

**Fig. 9.13:** Right (a), Left (b) middle meatal antrostomy being performed using a back biting forceps (BBF)

Care is taken not to open the ostium anterior to the level of the middle turbinate to prevent injury to the nasolacrimal duct.

## Exploration of the Frontal Recess and Frontal Sinusotomy

The frontal recess can be explored after the removal of anterior ethmoidal cells and bulla and identification of ethmoidal roof. An

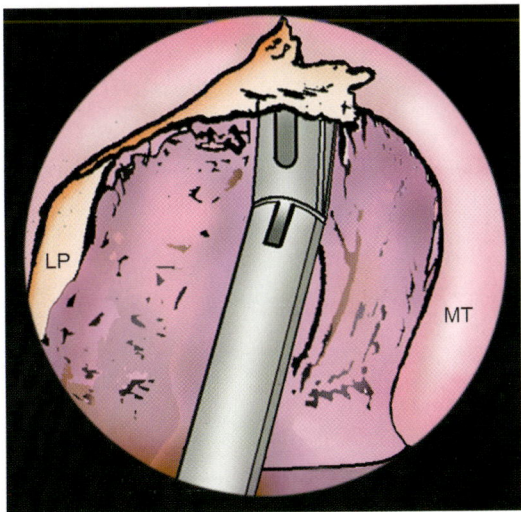

**Fig. 9.15:** Clearance of the frontal recess with Blakesly forceps

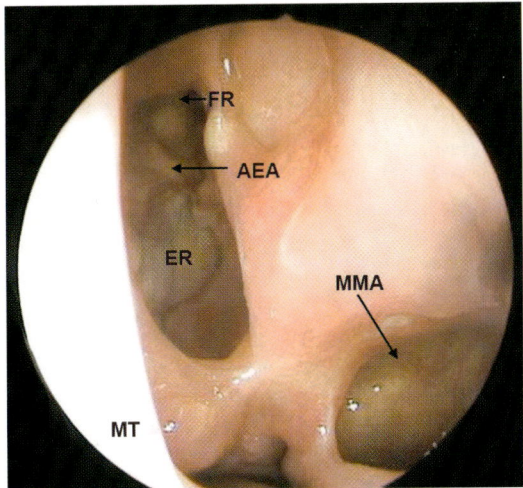

**Fig. 9.14:** Video endoscope picture showing the post-operative picture of ostium after middle meated antrostomy (left)

angled Blakesly forceps and 30° nasal endoscope are used for this purpose (Figs 9.15 to 9.17). As there are a lot of anatomical variations in this area, the exact technique varies. It is usually possible to view sinus after tracing the cranial extent of the uncinate process remnant on its posterior aspect. The superior attachment of the bulla should be preserved as frontal recess lies always anterior and superior to that. Incomplete removal of

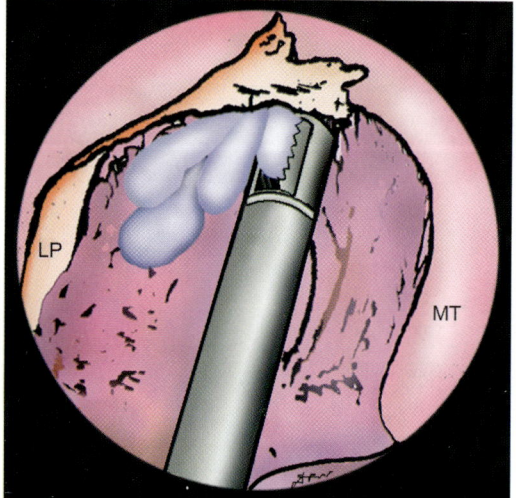

**Fig. 9.16:** Endoscope photograph showing polyp being removed from left frontal recess with microdebridor

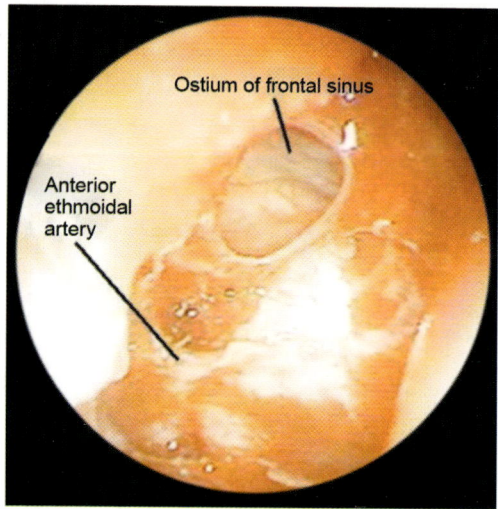

**Fig. 9.17:** Showing the frontal sinus ostium after clearance of the left frontal recess

cells or striping of mucosa is one of the causes for stenosis of the frontal ostium. Preoperative spiral multi slice CT is essential to analyze the anatomy of the frontal recess with the user friendly Kuhn's classification of frontal ethmoidal cells. A ball probe or a curved curette is an useful instrument to uncap and

exenterate the frontal and agger nasi cells and should be done from the posterior to anterior fashion under vision. At no stage a curette or the probe should pass through the roof of a cell. If the bulla is removed completely especially in the previous surgery (Fig. 9.14), the anterior ethmoidal artery is identified

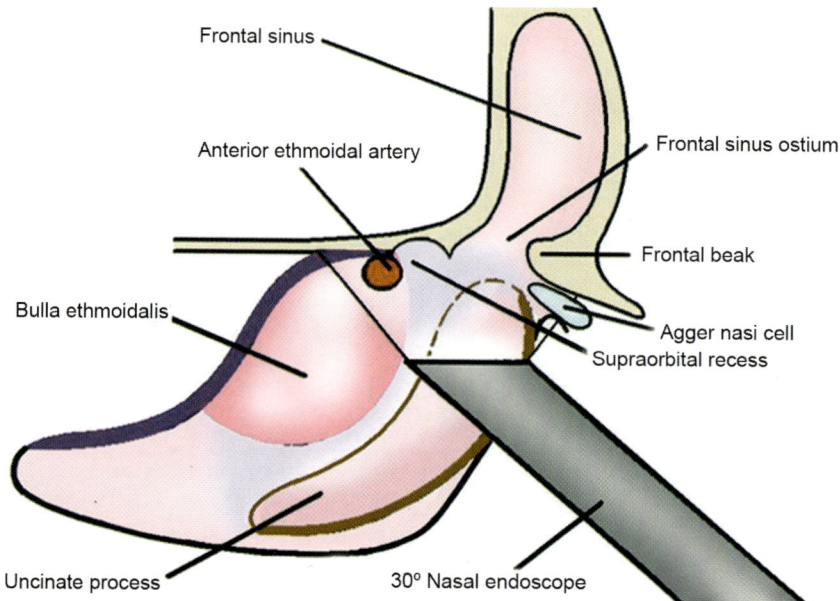

**Fig. 9.18:** Position of (1) supraorbital recess, and (2) frontal ostium

using the 30/70 degree scope to locate a small recess which usually opens into a supraorbital recess directly in front of the artery, and frontal ostium is further anterior (Fig. 9.18). Often there are difficulties in identifying the frontal ostium due to previous surgery or extensive disease in the frontal recess. It is often useful to raise an axillary flap described by Wormald 2002 similar to that for DCR of 7–8 square mm from lateral wall towards the middle turbinate to expose the anterior wall of the agger nasi. The anterior wall is then removed to identify the agger nasi cell by using a drill or Hajek-Kofler punch forceps (Fig. 9.19a). The agger nasi cell is carefully removed and other cells are identified. The frontal sinus drainage pathway is carefully identified with a curved ball probe.

The removal of frontal cells individually from posterior medial to anterior direction without injuring the attachment of the middle turbinate finally allows the visualization of the frontal ostium (Fig. 9.19b). Enlargement of the ostium is done anteriorly while taking care to preserve the mucosa. The axillary flap is placed into the cavity to cover the raw bony surface to maximize the healing (Fig. 9.19c). This completes draf 1 procedure.

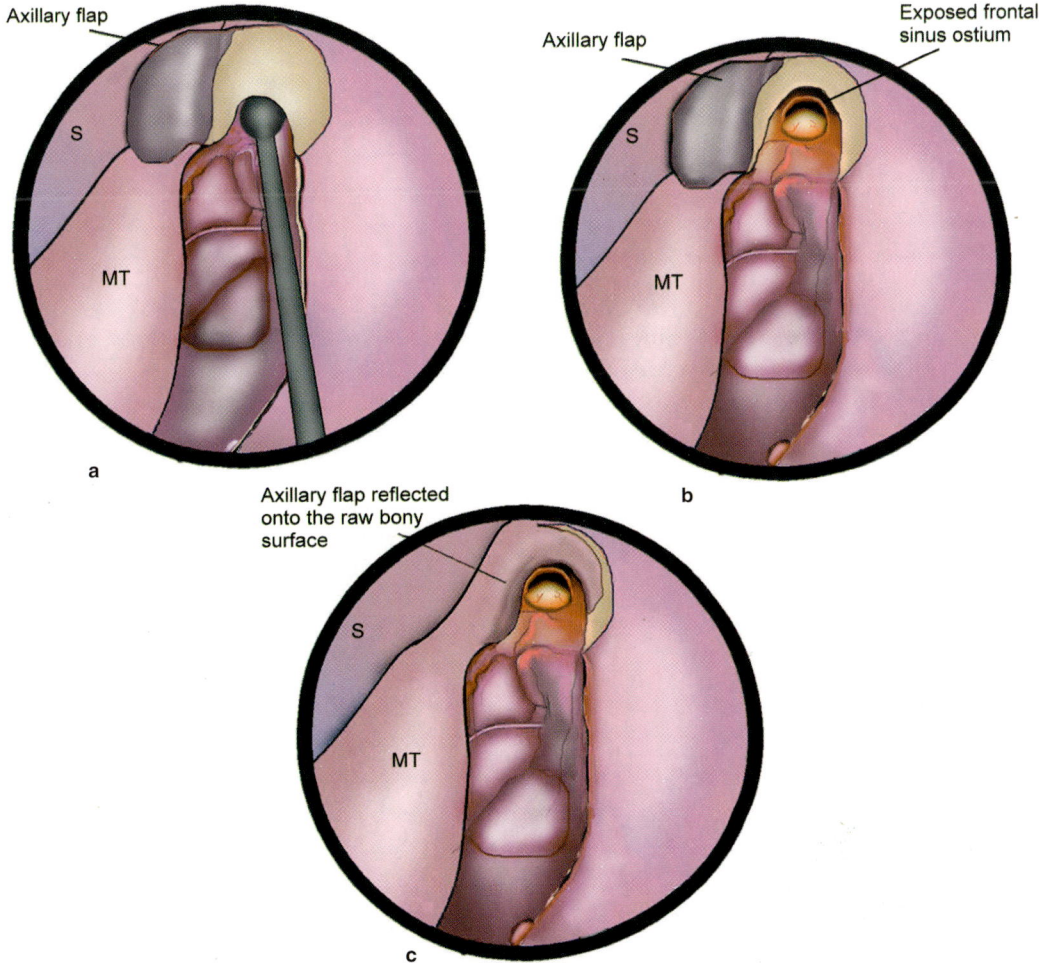

**Figs 9.19 a to c:** Showing (a) elevation and driling of anterior wall of agger nasi cell of axillary flaps, (b) excenteration of agger nasi air cell and removal of frontal cell to expose frontal sinus ostium (c) placement of axillary flap over raw bony surface

## Posterior Ethmoidectomy and Sphenoidotomy

In any operation on the posterior ethmoidal or sphenoid sinus, it is a must to study the tomograms preoperatively to analyze the spatial relationships between optic nerve, the internal carotid artery and the sphenoidal sinus. If the posterior ethmoid is diseased, the ground lamella is approached. Dehiscence and perforations of the ground lamella are the most common route through which disease spreads from anterior to posterior ethmoid. After ethmoidal bulla has been removed, the course of the ground lamella can easily be followed with the endoscope.

To open the posterior ethmoid, the ground lamella should be opened as far medially and inferiorly as possible. The best place is 3 to 4 mm cranially from the point where the ground lamella turns superiorly from its horizontal course as the roof of the posterior one third of the middle meatus, just behind the ethmoidal bulla (Figs 9.20 to 9.22). The entire ground lamella should never be removed totally as it can destabilize the middle turbinate. The larger cells and milder disease usually allow easy; skull base identification. If skull base cannot be identified as in extensive disease, it may be

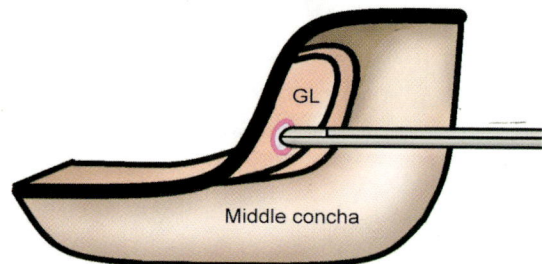

Fig. 9.21: Ground lamella being opened in its inferomedial aspect (after Stammberger)

necessary to open the sphenoidal sinus initially before skull base is identified. In a markedly pneumatized posterior ethmoids, the optic nerve can be seen posteromedially as a convexity in the wall of the posterior ethmoid sinus.

If the sphenoidal sinus need to be opened, the surgeon must remember that the path through the ethmoid does lead to the anterior wall of the sphenoid. The bulge of the sphenoidal sinus is evident in the inferomedial aspect of the most posterior ethmoid and should be opened under direct vision (Figs 9.23 and 9.24). The depth of penetration should also be measured using measuring probe or suction tip. Bulging of the optic nerve and internal

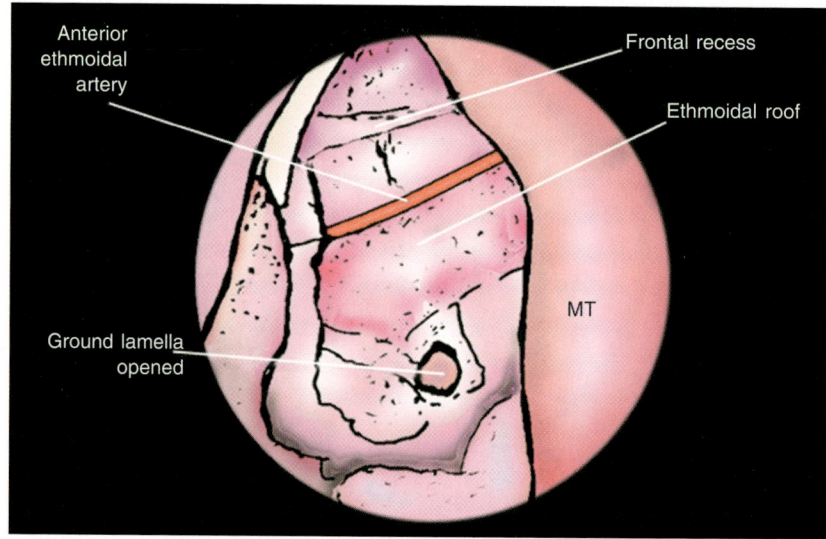

Fig. 9.20: Ground lamella being opened (right)

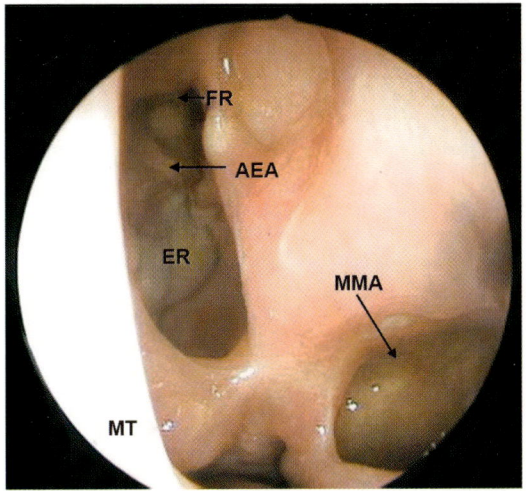

**Fig. 9.22:** The frontal recess, anterior ethmoidal artery and opening of posterior ethmoids. Maxillary ostium is seen laterally after middle meatal antrostomy on the left side. The cavity is well epithelialized postoperatively

carotid artery may be seen in the inferolateral aspect (Figs 9.25a and b) on a close-up view after opening the sphenoidal sinus.

As the dissection is performed from anterior to posterior direction, the surgeon will encounter four distinct bony laminas (Fig. 9.26). Identification and recognition of these landmarks during the dissection prevent the possibility of any intracranial and intraocular injury. In case of unfamiliar anatomy, previously operated case and for the beginner, a measuring probe should always be used to confirm the landmark. Bleeding is usually minimal under local anesthesia with proper vasoconstriction, and trauma to the turbinate and vascular lateral nasal wall is avoided.

## Wigand's Technique

This surgical approach is performed under hypotensive general anesthesia.

### The Steps of Surgery

1. Septal mobilization and partial middle turbinate resection.
2. Bipolar cauterization of sphenopalatine artery is required to control the bleeding.

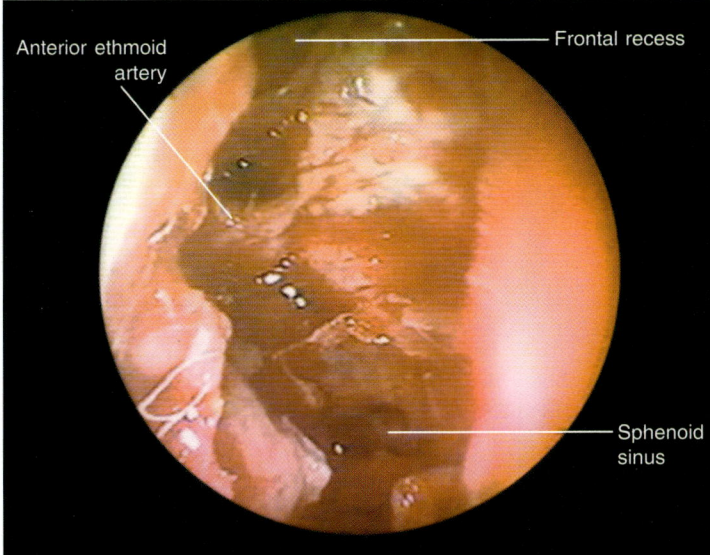

**Fig. 9.23:** Endoscopic photograph showing sphenoid being opened inferomedially after posterior ethmoidectomy on the left side

| Key for Figs 9.2 to 9.29 |
| --- |
| CM - Middle turbinate |
| PU - Uncinate process |
| LP - Lamina papyracea |
| BE- Bulla ethmoidalis |
| RE/ER - Roof of ethmoid |
| GL - Ground lamella |
| A - Anterior ethmoidal artery |
| Sp/Sps - Sphenoidal sinus |
| LN - Lateral nasal wall |
| S - Septum |
| PE - Posterior ethmoid |
| F - Frontal sinus |
| MS - Maxillary sinus |
| OMS - Ostium maxillary sinus |
| Adi - Additional lamella |
| FR/rf- Frontal recess |
| BBF - Back biting forceps of ostium of frontal sinus |
| ON - Optic nerve |
| ICA - Internal carotid artery |

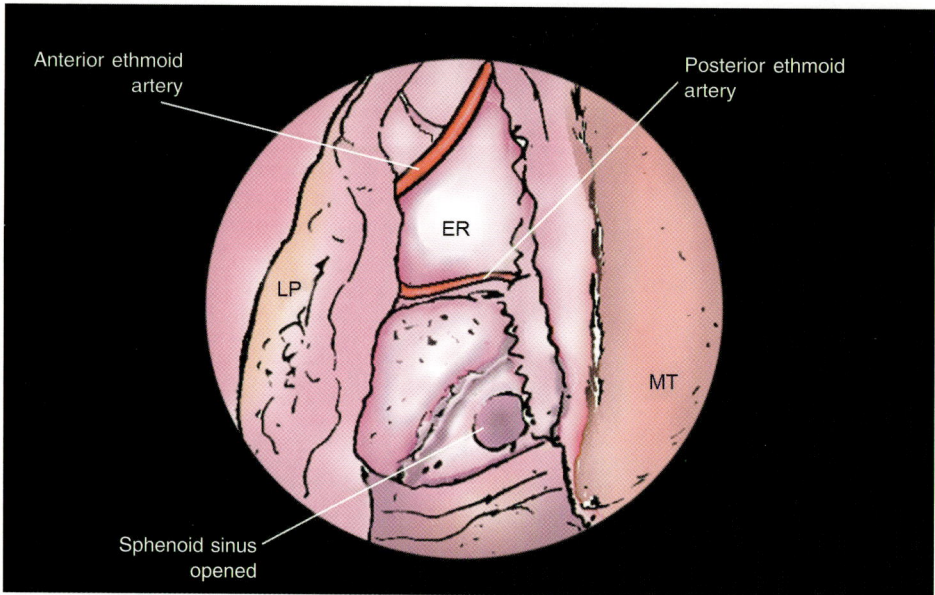

**Fig. 9.24:** Opening of the sphenoid inferomedially after complete ethmoidectomy on the right side

3. The medial position of posterior ethmoidal sinus is taken down under direct visualization through a headlight.

4. Sphenoid ostium is located.

5. Anterior wall of the sphenoid is removed.

6. The skull base is identified and the lateral wall of sphenoid is kept as landmark.

7. Dissection starts from that region towards a posterior anterior direction.

8. Agger nasi is removed for adequate visualization of frontal recess.

9. The 70° telescope is used to dissect the frontal recess and maxillary sinus.

10. A complete sphenoethmoidectomy is done.

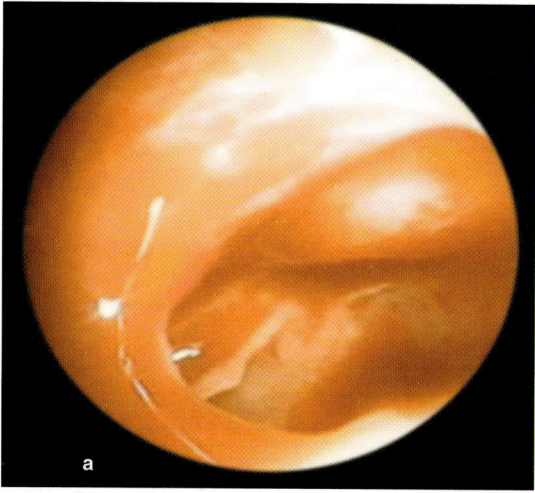
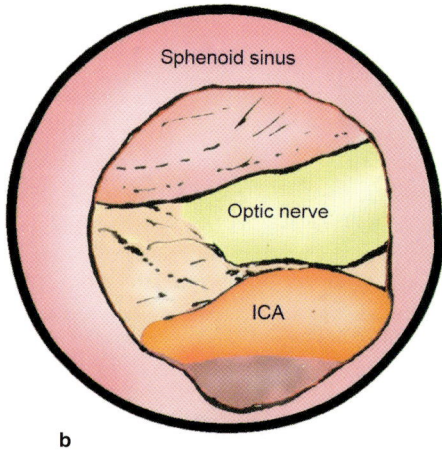

**Fig. 9.25: a.** Video endoscopic photograph showing optic nerve and internal carotid artery after sphenoid is opened (sphenoidotomy) **b.** Diagrammatic representation of the same

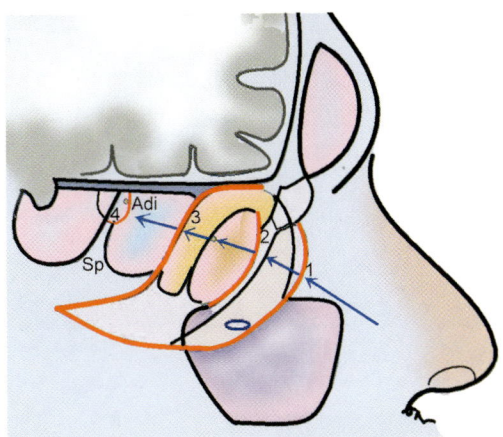

**Fig. 9.26:** Diagrammatic representation of the 5 lamellae that are encountered during an anterior to posterior dissection

## Endoscopic Management of Ethmoidal Polyposis and Antrochoanal Polyp

Functional endoscopic sinus surgery (FESS) can be used effectively as a minimally invasive technique. The endoscope is used to improve ventilation and drainage in addition to polyp removal as described already under Messerklinger's technique of endoscopic sinus surgery. The extent of surgery varies according to the extent of disease and surgeon's individual practice. Initially the steps include gross removal of polyposis with the help of a Luc's forceps or a microdebrider for proper visualization of middle meatus. Then the surgery is performed as done under conventional endoscopic sinus surgery with the help of a microdebridor (shaver). The endoscopic surgical technique has been used for more than a decade in treating sino-nasal conditions. Advantages include a better view of the surgical field, a more precise and thorough clearance of the inflammatory changes. The use of microdebridor gives added advantage of cutting and at the same time suctioning to facilitate clear field of vision which is required for safe and effective in getting functional outcome. The shaver was first applied in orthopedic surgery. In the field of ENT it was first used by Setliff (1994 and 1995). The shaver (powered instrument) system offer different handpieces, knives, irrigation and modes

(rotating or oscillating). Shaver is a combination of suction and cutting round knife working together. Knives of different shapes are put into handpiece. They have outer sheath with a window, which protects the inner rotating blade. The blade is connected to suction and cutting tissue is removed from the operation field. In otolaryngology surgery we mostly use the oscillation cutting mode which is the most sufficient. Shaver surgery is precise in soft tissue resection, so the most advantages to power the system is in rhino-surgery, polypectomy with extension to pansinus surgery (Dalke *et al.* 2006) (Figs 9.27a to 9.29).

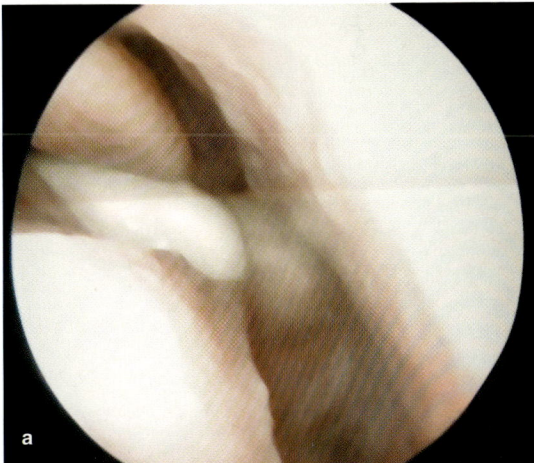

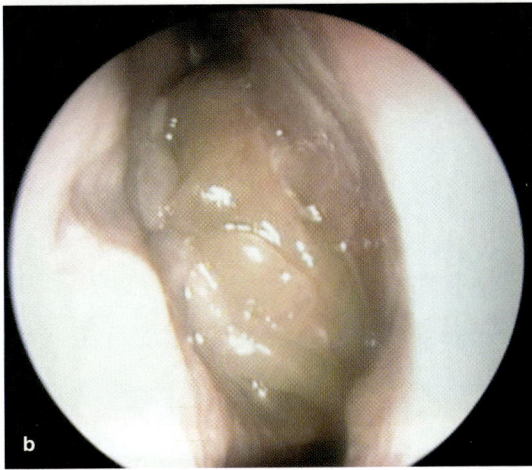

**Fig. 9.27: a.** Video endoscopic photograph showing right antrochoanal polyp, **b.** Left ethmoidal polyposis

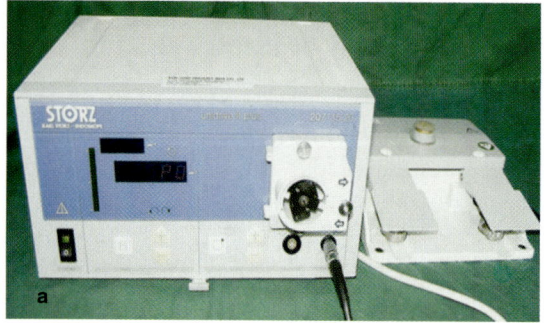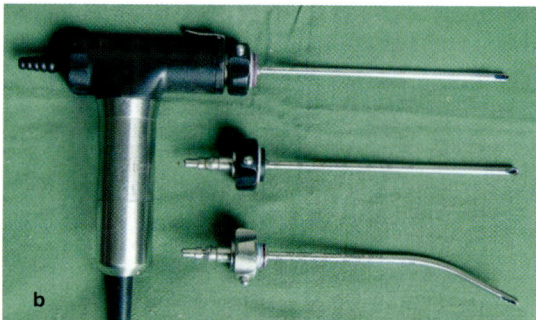

**Fig. 9.28: a.** STORZ microdebridor system, **b.** Handpiece and blades

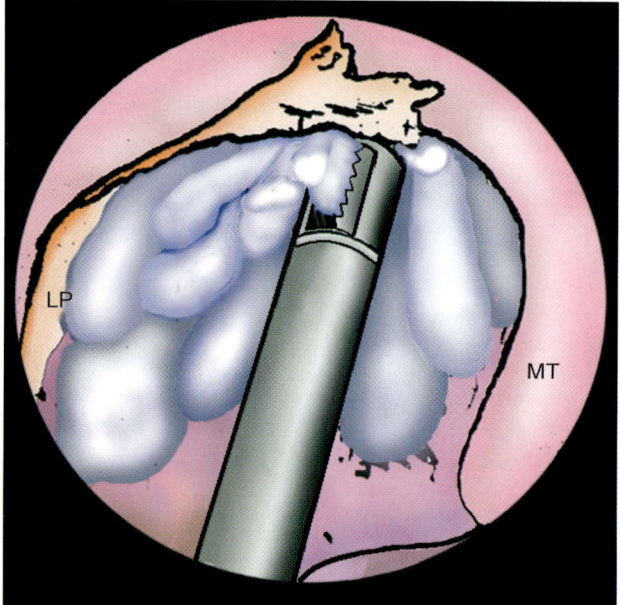

**Fig. 9.29:** Microdebridor assisted endoscopic sinus surgery for ethmoidal polyposis

The complications are few and recurrence rates are lower in comparison to conventional surgery in an experienced hand. The antrochoanal polyp is treated by using a forceps or a microdebridor to remove the polyp completely under endoscopic visualization from the antrum. Various types of angled handpieces are available for this purpose.

## Image-guided Endoscopic Surgery

Image-guided surgery has recently been described in the literature as a useful technology for improved functional endoscopic sinus surgery localization. Image-guided surgery yields accurate knowledge of the surgical field boundaries, allowing safer and more thorough sinus surgery. The InstaTrak system is used for this technique with excellent results. Computer-aided endoscopic sinus surgery appears to be the wave of the future. Nevertheless, the modern endoscopic sinus surgeon must have thorough training in the basic anatomy of the paranasal sinuses as well as the various surgical techniques. This technique is useful in revision cases extensive disease with distorted anatomy and endoscopic skull base surgery. A prior CT scan is taken, which are then processed and

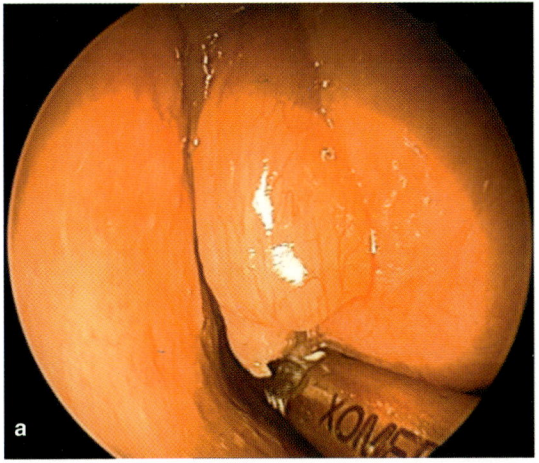
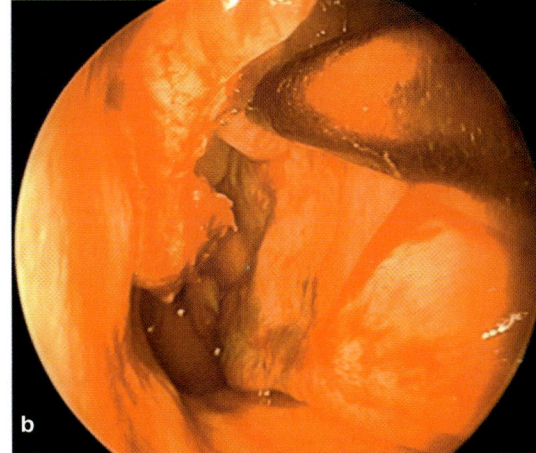

**Fig. 9.30: a.** Polyp arising from middle turbinate is being removed with microdebrider, **b.** middle turbinate is trimmed and the polypoidal tissue removed from the middle meatus to expose the uncinate process

downloaded onto the computer, where all the 2 sinus views (coronal, axial and sagittal) are displayed at the same time on the computer monitor. During surgery, the system is taken to the operating room and the same thing is viewed while the surgeon inserts a special probe in the nose that can be seen with standard surgical instruments.

### Uncinate Process Preservation Endoscopic Sinus Surgery

Nayak *et al*. (2001) were the first to introduce uncinate process preservation sinus surgery for patients having allergy associated rhinosinusitis. They found that limited endoscopic sinus surgery is more effective in managing postoperative problems than traditional FESS. This approach can also be used for patients having allergy associated ethmoidal polyposis (Figs 9.30a and b). Uncinate process is preserved while performing the maxillary sinusotomy and can be done without opening the bulla when ethmoid is not diseased. A small opening is created in the posterior fontanellae in the absence of an accessory ostium which is then communicated with the natural ostium. Diseased ethmoid is opened through a transbullar approach as done in FESS. Preservation of uncinate does not hamper clearance of frontal recess.

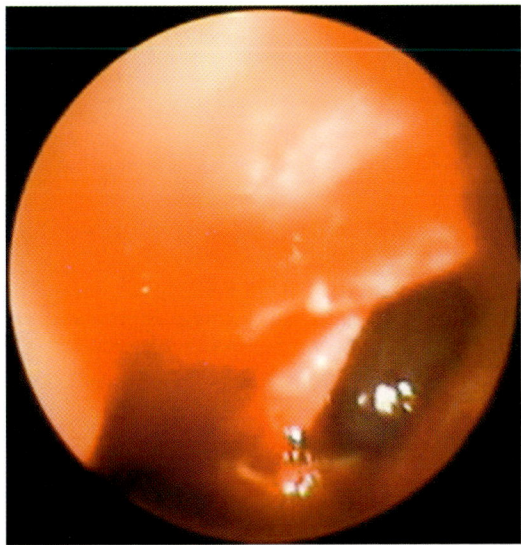

**Fig. 9.31:** Showing maxillary sinusostomy with intact uncinate process

Posterior ethmoidectomy is does in similar fashion. Middle turbinate trimming allows visualization of sphenoid ostium, that can be enlarged further using straight mushroom punch forceps. The author (DRN) terms the surgery functional endoscopic nasosinus surgery (FENS).

*Three-dimensional endoscopic sinus surgery:* Despite the progressive technological innovations in modern endoscopic surgery, the visualization that is currently used remains 2-dimensional (2D). The development of a miniature stereoscopic camera and its adaptation to rigid endoscopes allows for performance of 3D endoscopic sinus surgery. It is hypothesized that incorporation of 3D visualization may enhance the spatial resolution required in advanced endoscopic approaches with a theoretical potential to improve outcomes. Future applications of this technology include the ability to fuse an MR scan with the endoscopic picture to enable surgeons to have a view beyond that which is normally visible. These merged images will likely in the future be able to work with the next generation of image-guidance systems to allow surgeons to continue to expand minimally invasive surgery intracranially (Brown et al.).

## REFERENCES AND FURTHER READING

1. Stammberger Functional Endoscopic Sinus Surgery, BC Decker, Philadelphia 1991.

2. Kenedy D W. Functional Endoscopic Sinus Surgery Technique, Arch. Otolaryngology, 1985; 111:634.

3. MV Kirtane. Functional Endoscopic Sinus Surgery 1993.

4. Byron and Bailey. Head and Neck Surgery—Otolaryngology, (Ed) 1993.

5. W Messerklinger—Background and Evolution of Endoscopic Sinus Surgery. ENT 1994; Journal (73) 7449–55.

6. Stankiewicz JA. Complications in endoscopic ethmoidectomy: an update, Laryngoscope 1989; 99:686.

7. RC Setliff. New concepts and the use of powered instrumentation (the hummer) for functional endoscopic sinus surgery, in: JA Stankiewicz (Ed.), Advanced Endoscopic Sinus Surgery, Mosby, St. Louis, 1995, pp. 161–70.

8. RC Setliff, DS Parsons. The "Hummer": new instrumentation for functional endoscopic sinus surgery, Am. J Rhinnol. 8; 1994: 275–8.

9. Dalke et al. Rotation suction-knife (shaver) in otorhinolaryngological surgery. Otolaryngol Pol. 2006; 60(1):37–40 (ISSN: 0030–6657).

10. Fried, Marvin P MD, FACS et al. Image-Guided Endoscopic Surgery: results of accuracy and Performance in a multicenter clinical study using an Electromagnetic Tracking System. May 1997, Volume 107, Issue 5, 594 Laryngoscope. 107(5):594–601.

11. Anon, Jack B MD, FACS. Computer-Aided Endoscopic Sinus Surgery. 108(7):949–961, July 1998, Laryngoscope.

12. Nayak et al. Endoscopic physiological approach to allergy associated rhino-sinusitis. ENT Journal 2001, June 80(5):392–403.

13. Wormald PJ. The axillary flap approach to the frontal recess; laryngoscope 2002 March, 112(3):494–9.

14. Brown, et al. Three-dimensional endoscopic sinus surgery: Feasibility and technical aspects, Otolaryngology–Head and Neck Surgery, Vol 138, No 3, 40–42, March 2008.

# 10

# Postoperative Care

Postoperative care is one of the most essential aspect of endoscopic sinus surgery and is just as critical as preoperative assessment and the intraoperative technique, in preventing complications. The surgeon and the patient should both be fully committed to the postoperative cleaning and care including equipment inconvenience, discomfort and other factors required in achieving optimal results.

The most frequent and frustrating complication of functional endoscopic sinus surgery has been the tendency for scarring between the middle turbinate and the lateral nasal wall which leads to obstruction of the outflow at the osteomeatal complex as a result of synaechia formation. Other examples of unsatisfactory healing that would compromise results include recurrence of polyps, stenosis of sphenoid or maxillary ostium and frontal recess or perioperative infection. After functional endoscopic sinus surgery mucociliary function at the osteomeatal complex is impaired for approximately six weeks, until healing is complete. During this period, fibrosis, mucous secretion and blood clots tend to collect within the nasal cavity and osteomeatal complex area causing patient discomfort and predisposing to perioperative infection and/or scarring.

The plan for postoperative care begins during the preoperative consultation. In general, the timing of care is individualized. However, in our institute, we have found that the following timetable for postoperative care

is adequate for most patients. Usually the first postoperative cleaning is done on the 2nd postoperative day following surgery. The subsequent postoperative visits are after 1 week following surgery and then biweekly until the healing is complete which is usually by six weeks. Alternatively, particularly patient from far away place we advice saline irrigation after the first day of surgery and then endoscopic cleaning on postoperative day-2 and one week after. Thereafter, the patient is advised to follow aggressive saline irrigation with the help of a 10 cc disposable syringe. Postoperative nasal douching is common and evidence supports their efficacy in improving outcome following FESS, which may avoid the need for frequent office debridement (Tysome 2007). Postoperative use of nasal douching with hypertonic saline alone has shown comparable outcomes in terms of symptom scores and synechiae (Fernandes, 1999).

Patients whose occupations are not physically demanding may return to work within 2 days of surgery but physical exertion is inadvisable for 7 to 10 days after surgery. Patients are advised to avoid nasal irritants (fumes, excessive dust, etc.) until healing is complete. Patients may swim by 3 weeks after surgery but are advised against diving for 6 weeks postoperatively.

At the 1st postoperative visit the patient's nose is decongested and anesthetized by placing pledgets of 4% xylocaine and 1% phenylephrine in the nose. After 10 minutes, the pledgets are removed and any adhesion between the middle turbinate and the lateral wall are released. Crusts of fibrin, mucus or blood are removed by gentle suctioning. This relieves the headache and nasal obstruction experienced by a few patients in the early postoperative period. If adhesions are extensive, they are released and a wax plate is kept between the middle turbinate and lateral wall. At subsequent office visits similar local anesthesia and cleaning is again performed to remove loose crusts and clots. Aggressive debridement is avoided because it encourages bleeding and synechiae formation and delays healing. By 3 weeks the mucosa in the osteomeatal complex has usually healed. By the end of 6th week, the nasal mucosa begins to normalize and mucociliary flow has been re-established. At this point, a meaningful evaluation of symptomatic results can be obtained in most patients.

Much discussion has been made of the decision of whether or not to place intranasal packing immediately after endoscopic sinus surgery. Obviously, packing is required in cases of significant bleeding; however, in our experience overnight nasal packing is very rarely needed and is done especially in cases where septal surgery is done simultaneously. We at times use a temporary pack of cottonoids soaked in 4% xylocaine with 1 in 10,000, adrenaline which is placed within the osteomeatal complex and removed approximately 1 to 2 hours following surgery. We prefer a temporary pack if adequate homeostasis is to be achieved as the discomfort of packing and stagnation of secretions is avoided.

To prevent the frequent complication of synechiae or lateralization of middle turbinate various types of barriers are used within the osteomeatal complex. Various stents and packs including silicone sheets, gelatin film wrapped around gelatin foam, telfa sheets, septal splints with wax plates, antibiotic ointments and others are commonly used. We routinely use antiseptic antihemostatic gel and at times wax plate which is placed between the middle turbinate and lateral nasal wall and separate splint for septum if septoplasty has been performed in the same sitting (Nayak *et al.* 1995). This is a temporary barrier and is removed at the 2nd postoperative visit.

Stenosis of the maxillary ostium is occasionally seen in postoperative period. This is usually treated by enlarging the ostium under local anesthesia. Narrowing of the nasofrontal duct and inflammation in this area is treated by removing sites of inflammation. The same is true for the sphenoid ostium and residual ethmoidal cells.

Routine postoperative medications include antibiotics, decongestants, topical nasal (sprays) and systemic steroids. Topical steroids are used in the form of sprays over a period of about 6 months and sometimes more if there is associated nasal allergy. This is to prevent recurrence of polyps or edema of sinus mucosa.

Postoperative care is extremely important for a successful surgery and more so in the pediatric patient. Obviously children cannot tolerate the discomfort of postoperative care and hence every postoperative cleaning has to be done under general anesthesia. Therefore, children and parents are advised that endoscopic sinus surgery in children is a multistage procedure. Multistage procedure can be avoided if a splint like dental wax plate is used between the lateral wall and the middle turbinate (Nayak *et al.* 1998). Introduction of absorbable/bio-degradable packing materials like merogel, Nasopore (synthetic polyurethane), etc: soaked with antibiotic and steroid may overcome this problem in paediatric patient.

Aggressive postoperative care performed under local anesthesia in the office setting can greatly increase the success rate of this procedure and diminish the need to return to the operating room for revision endoscopic sinus surgery (Fig. 10.1).

The patient should strictly be advised to the following guideline

- Patient requires frequent return visits to the clinic for sinus cleaning over a period of four to six weeks until appropriate healing of the sinuses is achieved.

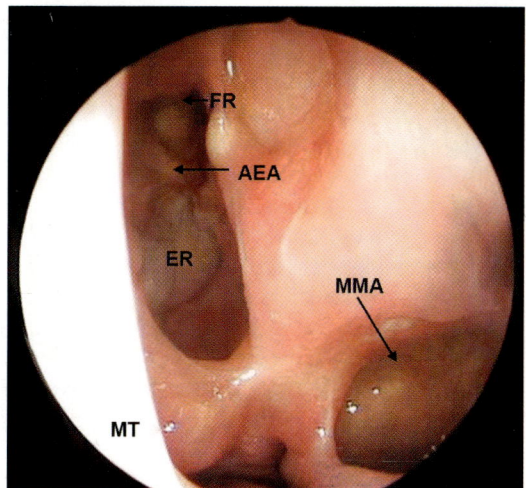

**Fig. 10.1:** Well epithelialized operated cavity after FESS, FR (frontal recess), AE (anterior ethmoidal artery), ER (ethmoidal roof), MMA (middle meatal antrostomy)

- Normal to have some bleeding for several days after surgery. If bleeding occurs, tilt your head back slightly and breathe gently through the nose.
- Should not blow the nose for one week following surgery and following the removal of splint or pack. After one week you may begin to blow your nose gently. Patient should sneeze with mouth open.
- For one to two weeks after surgery, use a saline nasal spray (non-decongestant) every 1–2 hours during the day to keep nose and sinuses moisturized.
- We prefer irrigation of homemade saline/ alkaline solution to flush the accumulated blood clots and crusts from the nasal cavity. Sinus should be rinsed twice a day following a day after surgery.
- Antibiotics like ciprofloxacin can be continued for several weeks after surgery.
- A dose of analgesic at least 45 minutes to one hour before the first postoperative cleaning is helpful.
- Patient should strictly be advised not to take aspirin or aspirin-related products.
- All strenuous activity should be avoided for at least two weeks.
- Some dark brown nasal discharge may be noticed several weeks after the surgery

that occurs as a result of old blood and mucus being cleared from the sinuses and is quite normal.

- Patient should consult the treating doctor as soon as possible if he experiences any of the following:
  - Watery nasal discharge (CSF leak)
  - Swelling of the eyes or diminished vision
  - High grade fever
  - Persistent headache
  - Neck stiffness
  - GI upset
  - Epistaxis

During the postoperative healing period, edema, crusting, secretions, and scarring are the major problems and need to be carefully managed to get a successful outcome after edoscopic sinus surgery. Postoperative nasal packing are often used to prevent postoperative hemorrhage and sometimes stent is used to prevent postoperative synechia formation and to facilitate better healing during this period. However, all these materials can cause severe discomfort to the patient and can be very painful on removal.

Jonnalagadda *et al*. 2011, found targeted topical pharmaceuticals have fewer side effect than systemic therapy and present an interesting option to treat chronic sinus disease. Techinque using bioabsorbable nasal sponges, such as Nasopore®, may introduce a fessible, safe, and effective methods of drug delivery, providing high concentrations of medication locally with lower sustainable concentrations systemically. Further study is necessary to elucidate the optimal concentration, dosing and effects.

Cote and Wright (2010) found a significant improvement in early postoperative healing in nasal cavities receiving triamcinolone-impregnated absorbable nasal packing following ESS and is also associated with improved healing up to 6 months postoperatively.

However, recent research shows promise with microporous polysaccharide hemospheres and chitosan gel having promising effects on hemostasis, and chitosan gel showing a significant adhesion prevention effect. The area of wound healing and adhesion prevention remains an area of active research and more prospective controlled trials are needed to define any benefits biomaterials may have (Rowan and Peter-John 2010).

The first author of this book (DRN) uses bio-degradable nasal packing like Nasopore® (polyganic) soaked with antinfective agent along with prednisolone to pack the ethmoidal cavity and also in the region sinus ostium and found encouraging results in achieving healing and prevention of synechia (Fig. 10.2).

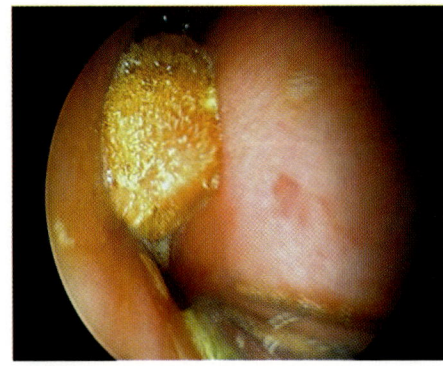

**Fig. 10.2:** Endoscopic picture showing Betadine and Triamcinolone shoked Nasopore® placed in the middle meatus and is left in situ while the patient is asked to irrigate the nose with normal saline at home

## REFERENCES AND FURTHER READING

1. Nayak, DR Balakrishnan R and Murty KD. Septal splint with wax plates". Journal of Postgraduate Medicine. "An endoscopic approach to deviated nasal septum—a preliminary study" 1995:41 (3); 70–71.

2. Nayak DR, Balakrishnan R and Murty KD. "Prevention and management of synechia in pediatric endoscopic sinus surgery using dental wax plates". International Journal of Pediatric Otolaryngology 1998: 46; 171–178.

3. Nayak DR, Balakrishnan R and Hazarika P. "An endoscopic approach to deviated nasal septum—a preliminary study". Journal of Laryngology and Otology 1998:112; 934–9.

4. Mair EA. Pediatric functional endoscopic sinus surgery: postoperative care. Otolaryngol Clin. North Am. 1996; 29 : 207–19.

5. Dipak Ranjan Nayak, Ramaswamy Balakrishnan, Deepak Murty K and Produl Hazarika. "Endoscopic septoturbinoplasty: our update series". Indian Journal of Otolaryngology and Head and Neck Surgery, 2002:54 (1):20–22.

6. Nayak DR, Balakrishna R and Murthy KD. Endoscopic Physiologic Approach to Allergy associated chronic rhinosinusitis—a preliminary study, ENT Journal 2001: 80(6):392–403.

7. Fernandes SV. Postoperative care in functional endoscopic sinus surgery; Laryngoscope 1999; 109:945–48.

8. Tysome JR, Sharp HR. Current Trends In Pre and Postoperative Management of Functional Endoscopic Sinus Surgery. The internet journal of otolaryngology 2007.

9. Cote DW and Wright ED. Triamcinolone-impregnated nasal dressing following endoscopic sinus surgery: a randomized, double-bline, placebo-controlled study. Laryngoscope. 2010 June; 120(6):1269–73.

10. Sashikanth Jonnalagadda, Vivian M. Yu, and Peter J. A feasibility Study to Evaluate a Novel Drug Delivery Technique through Nasal/Sinus Mucosa using a Biodegradable Polymer in a Guinea Pig Model. Catalano, Otolaryngology–2011 Head and Neck surgey 144(6):978–981.

11. Nasal dressings after endoscopic sinussurgery: what and why? Valentine rowan, Wormland; Current Opinion in Otolaryngology and Head and Neck Surgery: February 2010 Volume 18-Issue 1-p 44–48.

12. Rowan Valentine; Peter-John Wormald. Are routine dissolvable nasal dressing necessary following endoscopic sinus surgery? Laryngoscope 2010;120(12):2528–31.

# 11

# Complications of FESS

Since its introduction endoscopic sinus surgery has revolutionized the treatment of sinus disease. But with advent of its popularity the number of documented complications has also risen due to the intimate relation of sinuses to the orbit and anterior cranial fossa. Knowledge of the surgical anatomy by the endoscopic surgeon is absolutely essential to prevent complications. Even the most experienced surgeon may encounter problems. Stankiewicz (1989) in his first series of FESS patients, he reported a complication rate of 29% and in his second series he reported a complication rate of 2.2%. The incidence of major perioperative complications was 0.85%, with cerebrospinal fluid (CSF) leak being the most common.

The most common minor complications of ESS were those related to orbital penetration and middle turbinate adhesions; minor complications occurred in 6.9% (Levine *et al.* 1994). Despite advances in endoscopic sinus surgery technique and instrumentation, serious ophthalmic complications may still occur. Inadvertent entry into the medial orbital wall can result in ocular motility complications (Bhatti *et al.* 2001). The complications are characterized as:

## Major

- Hemorrhage
- Blindness
- Injury to internal carotid artery
- Cavernous sinus—ICA fistula
- Intracranial hemorrhage

- Pneumocephalus
- Brain abscess
- Death

## Minor

- Orbital hematoma
- Orbital surgical emphysema
- Nasolacrimal duct injury
- Antrostomy closure
- Synechiae

## HOW TO AVOID COMPLICATIONS

### Preoperatively

- Careful history of bleeding disorders
- Adequate medical treatment for chronic inflammatory conditions of paranasal sinuses before planning for surgery. This includes both antibiotics and steroids (local and/systemic).
- Ophthalmological examination including visual status of the patient.
- Proper outpatient endoscopic assessment prior to surgery.
- Preoperative CT scan is extremely important to assess the anatomical and pathological abnormalities which should ideally contain both axial and coronal cuts. The coronal cuts gives better information about anterior ethmoid, cribriform plate and frontal sinus in relation to the anterior cranial fossa, whereas axial cuts give more information about the posterior ethmoid, sphenoid and the orbit.

### Preoperatively

- Use of adequate decongestion before starting surgery is extremely important.
- As a beginner local anesthesia should be preferred over general anesthesia.
- 0 degree endoscope is the best to start with for a beginner.
- Angle endoscope should be avoided if the surgeon is not able to appreciate the landmarks properly. Absence of surgical landmarks like dehiscent lamina papyracea, radically resected middle turbinate, not able to identify maxillary ostium due to extensive disease or previous surgery are the potential risk factors for complications. In such situation a beginner should better avoid in attempting such cases. Such cases should be handled by surgeon having enough expertise. Preoperative CT scan is very useful in such cases. Recently CT guided surgery has been introduced to tackle such cases.
- The concept of surgery suggests limited surgery initially to anterior ethmoid, then posterior ethmoid and sphenoid as one gains confidence and finally the surgery for frontal recess should be tackled to prevent any major complication.

### Hemorrhage

Major bleeding points are anterior ethmoidal, posterior septal artery and the traumatized turbinate.

Packing usually controls bleeding. Cautery may be used judiciously.

Always terminate the surgery if the bleeding impairs visualization. Never operate in a bloody field. Pack, wait and then proceed.

### Synechiae (Figs 11.1 and 11.2)

Synechia is usually caused due to oppose raw surfaces of the middle turbinate and ethmoid cavity. Figure 11.1 is showing the synechia between inferior turbinate and septum and Fig. 11.2 showing early synechia between middle turbinate and lateral wall that may obstruct middle meatal drainage. Only 20% are symptomatic and requiring revision surgery. Symptoms include nasal obstruction, headaches

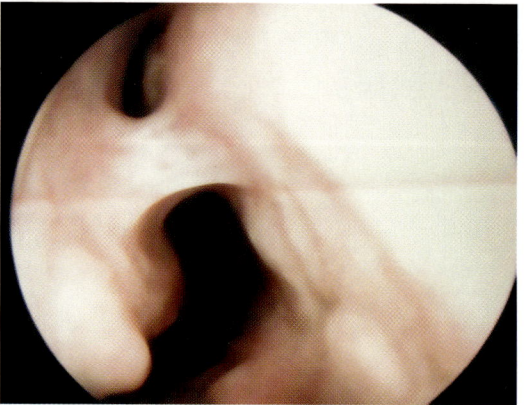

**Fig. 11.1:** Video endoscopic photograph showing synechia between septum and inferior turbinate

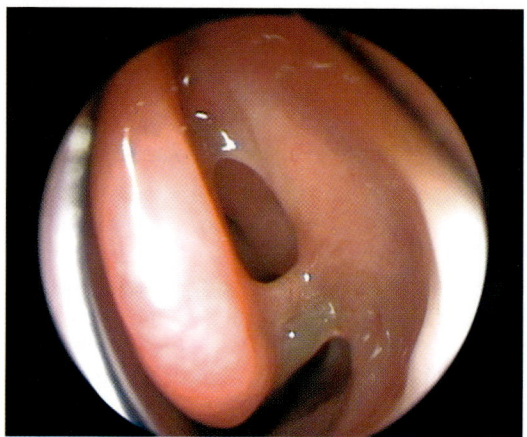

**Fig. 11.2:** Video endoscopic photograph showing synechia between middle turbinate and lateral nasal wall

and smell dysfunction. Nayak, et al. in 1998 classified this adhesive condition, based on their site and clinical presentation, into four different groups and advocated use of splint made up of wax plate to prevent this complication.

Partial amputation of the middle turbinate antero-inferiorly may prevent synechiae. Gel foam, merocel, etc. have been proposed as spacers. Most adhesions can be lysed in the early postoperative period during suction and cleaning.

### Middle Meatal Antrostomy Closure

This occurs in about 2% of cases. A circumferential removal of tissue during antrostomy will contribute to scarring and subsequent closure. However, a 3 mm diameter opening is thought to be adequate for physiological drainage.[3]

The suggested method currently is to open the antrostomy posteriorly anteriorly and inferiorly.[1] Frequent cleanings and irrigations may prevent closure. Middle meatal antrostomy stents have gained acceptance lately.

Recent use of steroid-eluting stent is effective in improving wound healing by preserving sinus patency, reducing inflammation, and minimizing adhesions via controlled local steroid delivery without measurable systemic exposure (Murr et al. 2011).

## Nasolacrimal Duct Injury

This occurs due to excessive enlargement of the anstrostomy anteriorly. Normally there is injury to the lacrimal bone found superiorly in the middle meatus.[4]

Preventive recommendations include enlarging the maxillary ostium posteriorly and inferiorly. Anterior dissection should be limited to the level of the anterior end of the middle turbinate.

## Periorbital Emphysema

Lid edema, ecchymosis and emphysema all indicate disruption of the lamina papyracea. Even in experienced hands, the incidence of orbital complications is at 0.5–1.5%.

These findings usually will resolve spontaneously in 1–2 weeks. Close observation of visual acuity and pressure is necessary.

The presence of yellow orbital fat prolapsing into the operative field along with transmitted movements on movement of the eyeball is almost pathognomonic. All tissues removed during the surgery should be placed in water-floating tissues normally indicate presence of fat.

## Retro-bulbar Hemorrhage

This is characterized by ecchymosis, proptosis, orbital pain, conjunctival hemorrhage. This is caused often due to injury to the anterior ethmoidal artery which retracts into the orbit and continues bleeding. An immediate lateral canthotomy is helpful (Dallan et al, 2009).

## Optic Nerve Injury

Direct injury to the optic nerve, in some cases bilaterally, has been reported in literature.[6]

Probable factors involved are inadequate visualization, poor understanding of anatomy and disorientation secondary to bleeding. 14% of patients have posterior ethmoid cells which extend over the sphenoid (Onodi cells). 88% of sphenoid sinuses juxtaposed the optic nerve and 23% of these had a significant bulge to the sphenoid. Knowledge, therefore, of the sphenoid and the posterior ethmoids is mandatory.

**Prevention of orbital complications is possible if the following guidelines are followed.**

Preoperative evaluation with regard to history of bleeding diathesis, aspirin use, hypertension, prolonged steroid use, glaucoma, visual activity, previous nasal surgery are extremely important.

Preoperative CT is important especially in patients with nasal polyposis and previous nasal surgery. Check for anatomical landmarks prior to surgery.

Keep the eyes uncovered after draping. Ask the patient to alert you in case of eye pain during the procedure, if under local anesthesia.

All tissues removed during surgery should be examined for orbital fat. Orbital ballotment may be necessary during the procedure to check for injury to the orbital periosteum.

Recognition of orbital hematoma is critical. Intranasal packs should be removed. Eye massage should be started immediately to redistribute the retro-orbital blood into the surrounding fat, thereby decreasing the orbital pressure.

Diuretics are given to decrease intraocular volume. Mannitol 1–2 gm/kg IV over 30 minutes to reduce intra-occular pressure, acetazolamide 500 mg IV reduces production

**Flow chart 11.1:** Orbital bleed/visual change algorithm

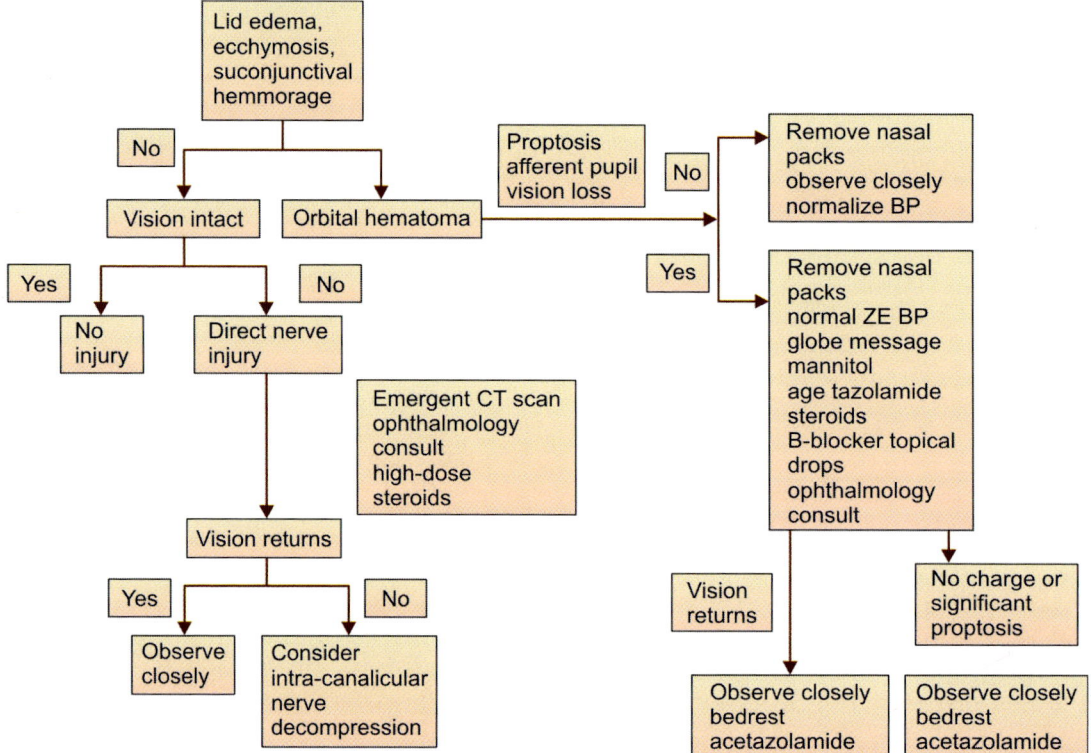

of aqueous humor, dexamethasone 10 mg IV bolus.[7]

If conservative management fails, then a lateral canthotomy with superior and inferior cantholysis will allow the orbit to expand.

A Lynch-Howarth approach with external ethmoidectomy and ligation of anterior and posterior ethmoid arteries will allow the periorbita to expand and help in the control of ocular pressure.

The intra-ocular pressure must be normalized within 98 minutes to prevent irreversible damage to the eye.[8]

### Cerebrospinal Fluid Leak

The incidence of CSF leak during FESS is reported at 0.05–0.9%. Leaks occur most often from the lateral lamella of cribriform plate, from the roof of the sphenoid or fovea ethmoidalis. Improper visualization, poor orientation, poor knowledge of anatomy, extensive polyposis and anatomical aberrations may cause these accidents. Kero's classification of olfactory fossa is a helpful guideline for the surgeon while dealing with the ethmoidal roof. Kero's type-3 has the highest risk for intracranial entry.

Prevention of this complication is the best arrangement. Intraoperatively, the leak can be plugged with temporalis fascia, fat or muscle. Postoperative leaks usually close spontaneously-advise the patient to avoid nose blowing, keep the head elevated, no lifting, bending or straining and absolute bedrest for 48 hours. A lumbar CSF drain may be required in some persistent leaks. If the leak persists in spite of a drain, then an endoscopic repair is advisable as described in Chapter 17. Larger defect requires anterior craniotomy for repair with 3 layer closure including sealing the bony defect.

## REFERENCES AND FURTHER READING

1. Thomas Neuman, WJ Turner, TM Davldson. Complications of Endoscopic Surgery. ENT 1994; Journal 73 (8):585–90.

2. Stankiewicz JA: Complications of Endoscopic Sinus Surgery. Otolaryngol. Clin North Am 1989, 22 (4): 749–58.

3. Hollmstead, WH. Anatomy for surgeons, The Head and Neck. JB Lippincott, Philadelphia. 1982, 93–158.

4. WE Bloger, Parsons DS, Mair TEA et al. Lacrimal drainage system injury in endoscopic sinus surgery. Incidence, analysis and prevention. Arch Otolaryngol 1992, 118(11): 1179–84.

5. Stankiewicz J. Complications in endoscopic intranasal ethmoidectomy: an update. Laryngoscope 1989: 99: 686–90.

6. Manlglla AJ. Fatal and other major complications of endoscopic sinus surgery. Laryngoscope 1991, 101: 349–54.

7. Stankiewicz JA. Blindness and intranasal endoscopic ethmoidectomy: prevention and management. Otolaryngol Head Neck Surg. 1989 : 101: 320–9.

8. Hayreh SS, Weingeist TA. Experimental occlusion of the central artery of the retina: retinal tolerance time to acute Ischemia. British Jour Ophthalmol 1980, 64: 818–25.

9. Dallan, et al. Management of severely bleeding ethmoidal arteries. J Craniofacial Surgery 2009, March, 20(2):450–4.

10. Abridged from Nueman, Turner, Davidson. Complications of Endoscopic Surgery. ENT August 1994; Journal Vol 73; 8: 585–90.

11. VJ Lund, A Wright, and J Yiotakis J. Complications and medicolegal aspects of endoscopic sinus surgery 1997 R Soc Med. August; 90(8): 422–428.

12. Levine HL, *et al.* Complications of endoscopic sinus surgery: analysis of 2108 patients-incidence and prevention. Laryngoscope. Sep; 1994 104 (9): 1080–3.

13. Bhatti MT *et al.* Ocular motility complications after endoscopic sinus surgery with powered cutting instruments, Otolaryngol Head Neck Surg. 2001 Nov; 125 (5): 501.

14. Keros PJ Laryngology Rhino et al. 1962, 41:809–13.

15. Lynch RC. The technique of radical frontal sinus operation which has given the best results. Laryngoscope 1921;31:1–5.

16. Nayak DR, et al. Prevention and management of synechia in pediatric endoscopic sinus surgery using dental wax plates. International Journal of Pediatric Otorhinolaryngology, 1998, Vol. 46, Issue 3, Pages 171–178.

17. Murr AH, et al. Safety and efficacy of a novel bioabsorbable, steroid-eluting sinus stent ; Int. Forum Allergy Rhinology 2011 Jan–Feb;1(1):23–32.

# 12

# Chronic Sinusitis—Management

*Dr R Singh*

## Definition

Chronic inflammation of the mucosal lining of one or more paranasal sinuses, usually caused by anatomical/pathological obstruction to its drainage, and is characterized by chronic postnasal mucopurulent discharge with or without recurrent headache/facial pain (more than 1 month) (Fig. 12.1).

## Type

- Open/close
- Unilateral/bilateral
- Single sinus/multisinusitis/pan-sinusitis

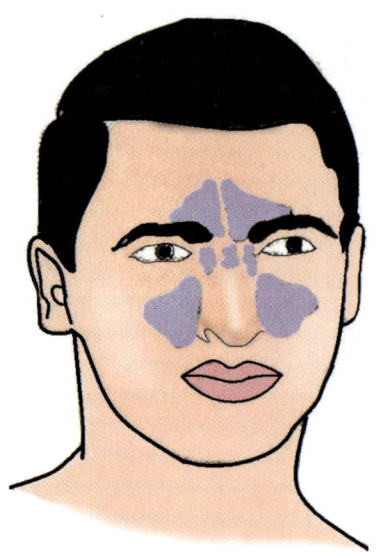

**Fig. 12.1:** Anatomical position of the anterior group of paranasal sinuses

- Anterior group/posterior group
- Suppurative/hypertrophic

## Etiopathogenesis (Flow chart 12.1)

- Usually rhinogenic. Other routes—rare.
- Unresolved acute sinusitis
- Any form of rhinitis → mucosal edema in OMC → pathological obstruction
- Any anatomical variation → anatomical obstruction
- Stagnation and secondary chronic sinusitis
- Mucosal edema
- Mechanical obstruction (anatomical)
- Mucous—thick
- Primary mucociliary dysfunction
- Anterior ethmoids is the key area for causation of chronic anterior group sinusitis because osteomeatal complex is situated within it, acts as a reservoir of infection.

## Bacteriology

- Mixed infection
- *Streptococcus pneumoniae, Streptococcus haemolyticus, Staph. aureus,* gram-negative bacteria, etc.
- Anaerobic infections cause fowl smelling discharge

## Pathology

- Open/closed type
- Mucosal changes

- Hyperemia
- Hypertrophy
- Increased mucosal glands
- Polypoidal changes
- Mucopurulent secretions
- Microabscesses
- Fibrosis, hyalinization
- Atrophy, squamous metaplasia, granulations

## Clinical Features

### Symptoms

- Mucopurulent/purulent postnasal discharge
- Cachosmia in case of anaerobic infection
- Headache/facial pain—depending on the site and type—usually dull aching.
- Nasal obstruction
- Aural and throat symptoms

### Signs

- Discharge in the middle meatus (MM) on anterior rhinoscopy
- Mucosal changes in the MM
- Discharge in MM/superior meatus (SM) on posterior rhinoscopy
- Tenderness in acute exacerbations
- Postural/transillumination tests
- Prominent lateral pharyngeal band

### Investigations

- Plain radiographs Water's view
- Mucosal thickening, haziness, opacity, polyp
- CT scan of OMC/paranasal sinuses (coronal cuts) (Figs 12.2a and b)
- X-ray nasopharynx in children to rule out enlarged adenoid
- Diagnostic nasal endoscopy

**Flow chart 12.1:** Pathogenesis of chronic sinusitis

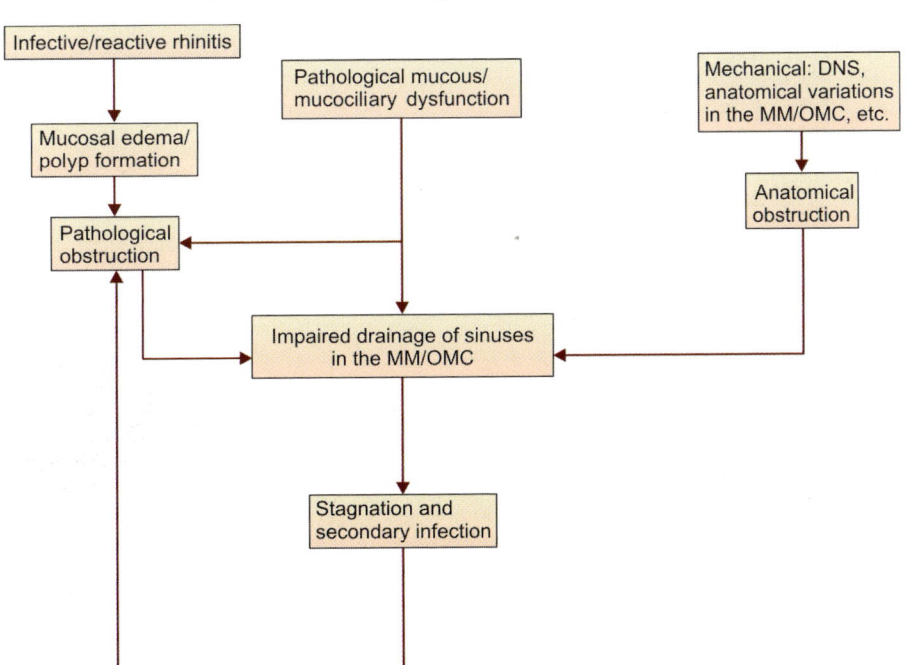

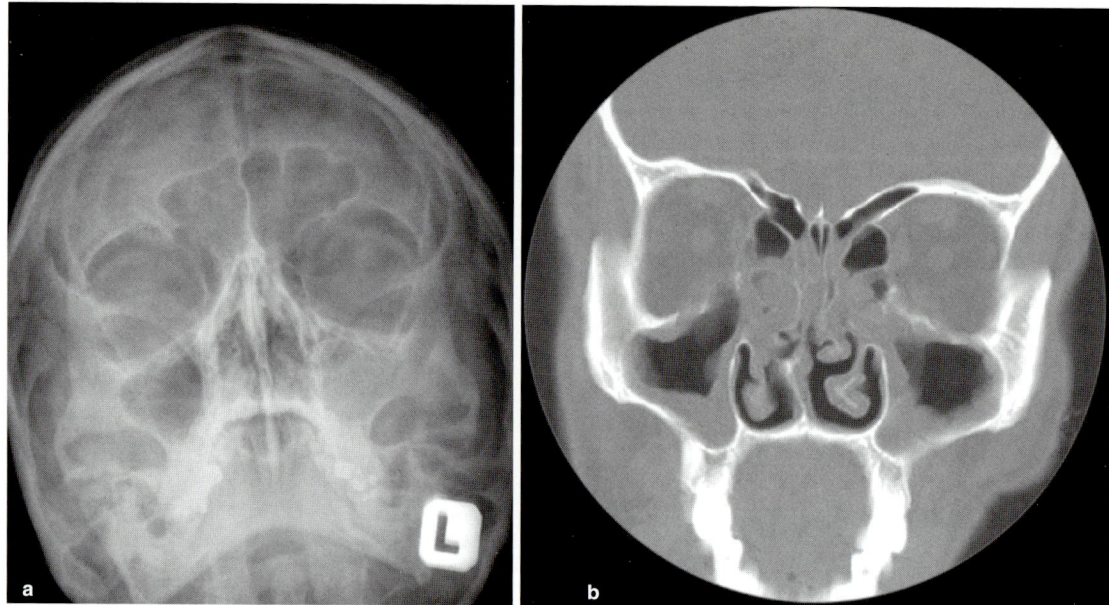

**Figs 12.2a and b:** X-ray PNS and CT OMC coronal cuts suggestive of bilateral OMC disease

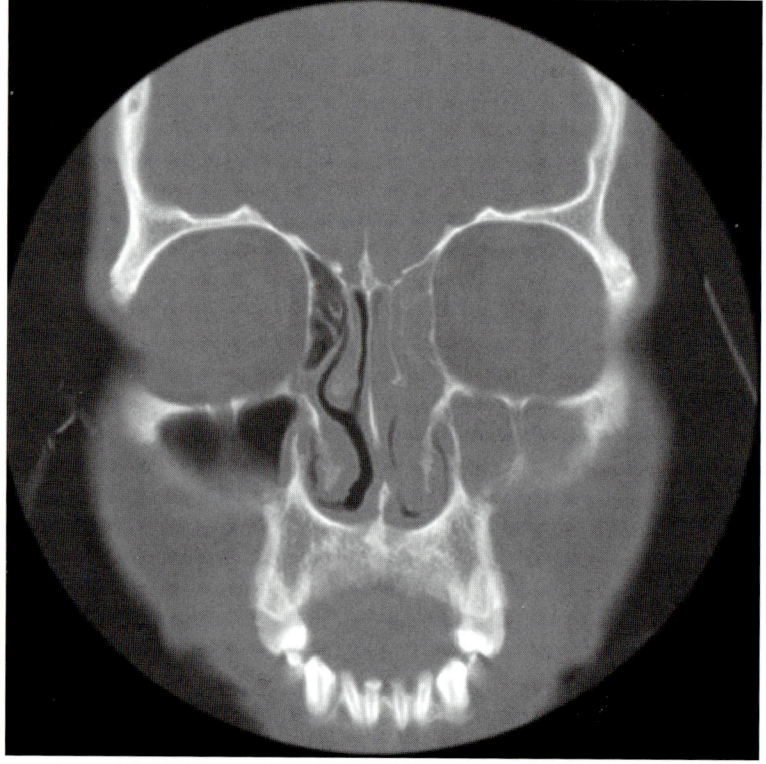

**Fig. 12.3:** CT OMC coronal cuts left pan sinusitis

- Allergic tests if suspected for nasal allergy
- Proof puncture for maxillary sinus
- Culture and sensitivity—rarely done
- Fungal culture of cheesy discharge, if present.

## Treatment

### *Medical*

- Antibiotics
- Nasal decongestants topical/systemic
- Antihistaminic
- Analgesics and anti-inflammatory
- Medicated steam inhalation
- Alkaline nasal douches
- Steroid nasal spray/short course of systemic steroids
- Antiallergy treatment

### *Surgical*

- When refractory to medical treatment
- Surgery for predisposing causes like DNS, polyp, etc.
- Surgical procedure depends on the sinus involved

- All sinuses may be surgically accessed endoscopically. CT guided endoscopic surgery helps in identifying various important landmarks like knowing the level of cribriform plate during surgery thus reducing major complications (Figs 12.4 and 12.5). Knowing this Kero's classifications of olfactory fossa is important for a surgeon.

The coronal CT allows to study the level of the cribriform plate and the olfactory fossa as described by Kero. This includes—(a) Kero's Type-1: olfactory fossa 1–3 mm deep, Type-2: olfactory fossa 4–7 mm deep, Type-3: olfactory fossa 8–16 mm deep (Fig. 12.5).

## Surgical Options for Chronic Maxillary Sinusitis

- Antral puncture
- Intranasal antrostomy
- Endoscopic middle meatal antrostomy (MMA) (Fig. 12.6)
- Endoscopic inferior meatal antrostomy (IMA) as shown in Fig. 12.7
- Caldwell-Luc operation (Fig. 12.8)
- Balloon sinuplasty

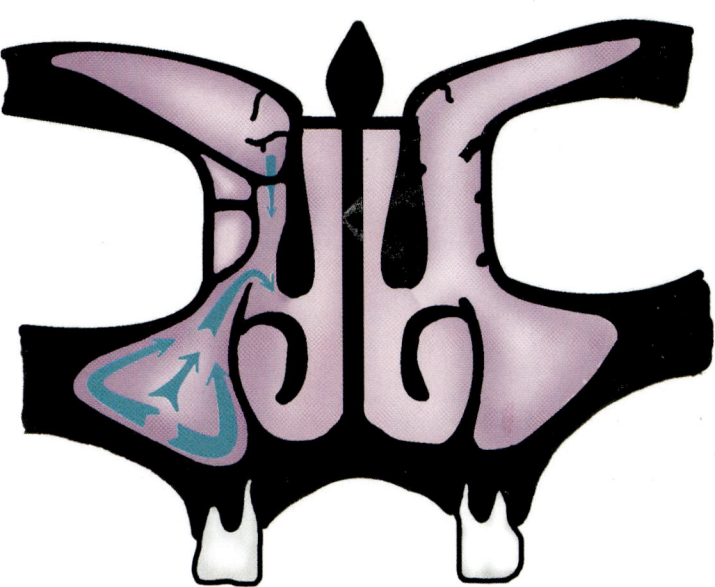

**Fig. 12.4:** Pre- and postendoscopic sinus surgery

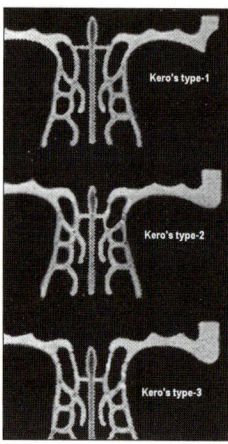

Fig. 12.5: Level of cribriform plate as described by Kero

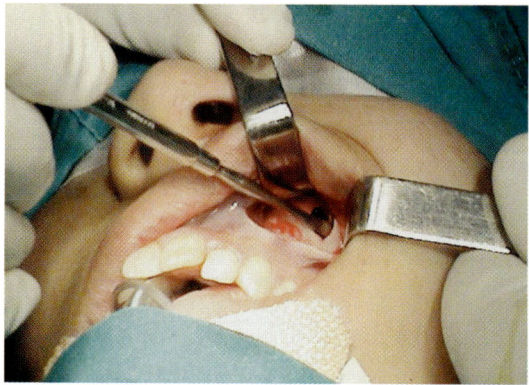

Fig. 12.8: Caldwell-Luc operation

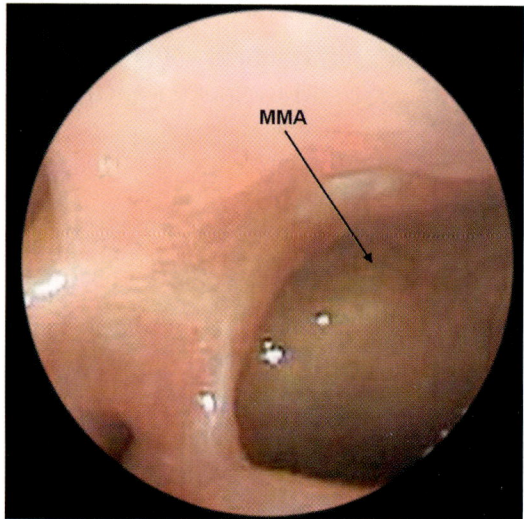

Fig. 12.6: Middle meatal antrostomy (MAA)

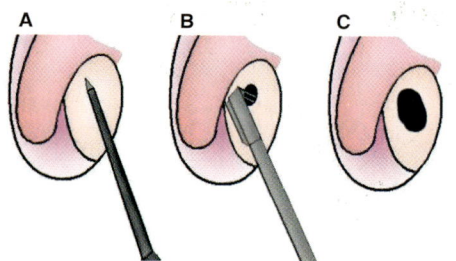

Fig. 12.7: Procedure of endoscopic inferior meatal fenestration (antrostomy)

## Chronic Ethmoiditis

- **Intranasal ethmoidectomy**
  - Complication—blindness
  - Dangerous procedure
- **Trans-antral ethmoidectomy**
  - Via Caldwell-Luc operation
- **External ethmoidectomy** (Howarth operation)
- **Endoscopic ethmoidectomy** (FESS)

## Chronic Frontal Sinusitis

- Balloon sinuplasty
- External fronto-ethmoidectomy (Lynch-Howarth operation)
- Osteoplastic operation
- Obliteration of frontal sinus
- Endoscopic frontal sinusotomy (Draf 1 and 2): In draf 2, frontal ostium is widened medially and laterally; besides removal of the frontal beak.
- Modified luthrop procedure (Draf 3): Involves drilling of the frontal sinus floor and resection of superior nasal septum and inferior interfrontal septum.

## Chronic Sphenoidal Sinusitis

- Intranasal sphenoethmoidectomy
- External sphenoethmoidectomy
- Endoscopic sphenoidotomy
- Balloon sinuplasty

## Steps for Functional Endoscopic Sinus Surgery

- Uncinectomy (infundibulotomy)
- Middle meatal antrostomy
- Frontal recess clearance
- Anterior ethmoidectomy
- Posterior ethmoidectomy
- Sphenoidotomy (Figs 12.9 and 12.10)

*Conclusion*

- Osteomeatal complex (OMC) disease is responsible for chronic persistent sinusitis
- Functional endoscopic sinus surgery (FESS) is the treatment of choice for the management of chronic sinusitis

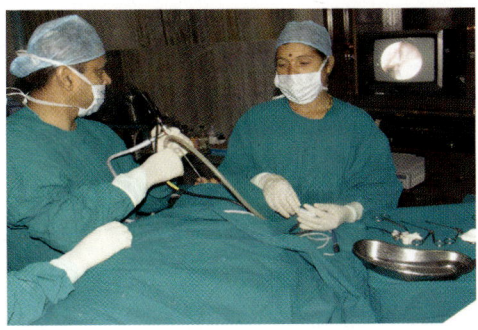

**Fig. 12.9:** Endoscopic sinus surgery in progress

- Meticulous postoperative care is the key to the success of endoscopic sinus surgery.

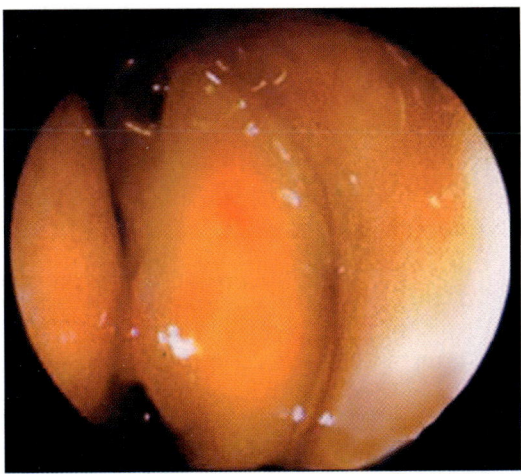 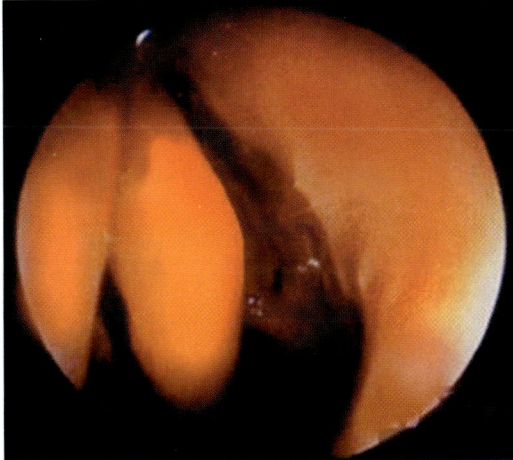

**Fig. 12.10:** Preoperative osteomeatal disease and ethmoidal cavity after endoscopic sinus surgery

## REFERENCES AND FURTHER READING

1. Stammberger. Functional Endoscopic Sinus Surgery, BC Decker, Philadelphia; 1991.
2. Kenedy DW. Functional Endoscopic Sinus Surgery Technique, Arch. Otolaryngology, 1985; 111:634.
3. Functional Endoscopic Sinus Surgery Dr MV Kirtane, 1993.
4. Head and Neck Surgery—Otolaryngology, Edited by Byron and Bailey (1993).
5. W Messerklinger. Background and Evolution of Endoscopic Sinus Surgery. ENT Journal 1994; (73) 7: 449–455.
6. Stanklewicz JA (1989). Complications in endoscopic ethmoidectomy: an update, Laryngoscope 1989; 99: 686.
7. John Groves, Roger F. Gray. A synopsis of Otolaryngology, 4th Edition, 1985.

# 13

# Endoscopic Septoturbinoplasty

Decades have passed since septoplasty was first introduced for the management of nasal airway. Numerous medical descriptions are available regarding the pathology and treatment of deviated nasal septum (Freer, 1902; Metzenbaum, 1929; Galloway, 1946; Cottle *et al.* 1958; Maran 1974).

The submucus resection was popularized and refined by Killian (1904) and Freer (1902). Due to the increased incidence of complications following such radical surgeries led to more and more conservative septal surgery. Metzenbaum 1929, described the swing-door technique for caudal dislocation and subluxation. Galloway (1946) removed the entire septal cartilage and replaced it as a separate autograft. Cottle (1958) described premaxilla-maxilla approach for the correction by making inferior and superior tunnel on concave side and inferior tunnel on convex side to facilitate necessary resection of cartilage and bone to correct the septal deformity. Maran (1974) has described septoplasty, but used a more radical technique in the terms of removal of bony septum. However, none of these descriptions have highlighted a complete surgical management of this condition to improve the nasal airway. Each surgical procedure has its limitations and cannot deal with all the variants of the deformities of the nasal septum. It is essential to know the biomechanical behavior of the cartilaginous septum (*Murakami et al. 1982*). Use of this technique has helped us to refine our technique of endoscopic septal correction. An ideal surgical correction of the nasal septum should satisfy the following criteria:

1. Should relieve the nasal obstruction.
2. Should be conservative.
3. Should not produce iatrogenic deformity.
4. Should not compromise the osteomeatal complex.
5. Should relieve all the contact areas.
6. Must have the scope for a revision surgery, if required later.

The traditional surgeries of the nasal septum improve the nasal airway but do not fulfill the above-mentioned criteria in most instances. The reasons outlined for this are poor visualization. Relative inaccessibility, poor illumination, difficulty in evaluation of the exact pathology, need for nasal packing, unnecessary manipulation, resection and over exposure of the septal framework, reducing the scope for a revision surgery (Nayak *et al.* 2002). The nasal endoscope allows precise preoperative identification of the septal pathology and its associated lateral nasal wall abnormalities and helps in better planning of endoscope-aided septal surgery (Nayak *et al.* 1998). This technique is ultra-conservative and fulfills the above mentioned criteria of an ideal septal surgery. As this surgery addresses both the septal and the turbinate pathologies, the term Endoscopic Septoturbinoplasty has been used by Nayak *et al.* (2002). In their preliminary study (1998), they demonstrated that endoscopic-aided approach in the management of deviated nasal septum, both subjectively and objectively is superior to the traditional technique. Simultaneous sinus surgery can be done without the fear of lateralization of the middle turbinate and consequent synechiae formation. Giles *et al.* (1994) in their series of 38 patients described the use of nasal endoscope in limited septal resection to facilitate endoscopic sinus surgery.

## Steps of Endoscopic Septoturbinoplasty
(Nayak *et al.* 1998, 2001 and 2002)

1. Surface anesthesia-4% xylocaine with adrenaline 1 in 100,000 for about 10 minutes.

2. Endoscopic infiltration of the nasal septum with 1 in 200,000 xylocaine with adrenaline on the convex side of the cartilaginous septum along the crest and bony septum on both sides including the spur whenever present.

3. Incomplete incision at the caudal end of the septum in its lower half in most cases except when there was a caudal dislocation or anterior buckling (hemi-transfixion).

4. Incision is made on the convex side in case with anterior deviation and on the concave side for subluxation, spur or posterior deviation to expose the abnormality at the bony cartilaginous junction. In cases of an isolated spur, incision is made parallel to the floor on the spur itself.

5. Elevation of the initial mucoperichondrial flap using Cottle's elevator and Pilchards nasal speculum. Further elevation is done using 0° Hopkins rod nasal endoscope (4 mm) held in left hand, keeping the tip of the endoscope between the mucoperichondrial flap and the septal cartilage. The right hand is used for instrumentation. Flap elevation in the correct cleavage plane is required to minimize bleeding. The exposure is limited to the target area. The traditional anterior and inferior tunnels described by Cottle *et al.* (1958) not followed in the endoscopic method.

6. A subluxated cartilage from the crest is shaved using no. 15-blade Bard-Parker knife to resect the excess cartilage inferiorly, without dislocating the vomero-chondral junction. At the anterior nasal spine, the subluxated cartilage was carefully trimmed and repositioned over the crest to prevent a supra-tip deformity (Figs 13.1a to d).

7. In case of posterior deviation or a deviation at the ethmo-chondral junction, the bony septum is fractured to realign in the midline or a minimum resection of the caudal end of the ethmoidal plate is performed. Dislocation of the ethmo-chondral junction should be avoided; especially in a child and a deviated septum here is precisely shaved using the Bard-Parker knife. However, a wedge resection can be performed after shaving the thick cartilage at the bony cartilage-nous junction in adults (Figs 13.2a and b).

8. A 'C'-shaped cartilaginous deviation is dealt with by precise multiple wedge resections on the convex side or multiple criss-cross incisions on the concave side aided by the endoscope, placing them on strategic sites and planes (as shown in Fig. 13.1).

9. In cases with caudal dislocation or anterior buckling of the cartilage the correction is done last after correcting the rest of the septum anticipating further increase in the anteroposterior length of the septum.

10. A spur without any other deviation of the septum is resected after incision and exposure made directly over the spur.

11. The gross anterior deviation is dealt with using traditional technique to start with and then treating the posterior deviation and the strategic central portion with the endoscopic approach.

12. A thick septum involving the posterior segment require precise shaving of the cartilage close to the bony cartilage junction and resection of the part of the vomer and perpendicular plate of the ethmoid if found thick (Figs 13.2a to d).

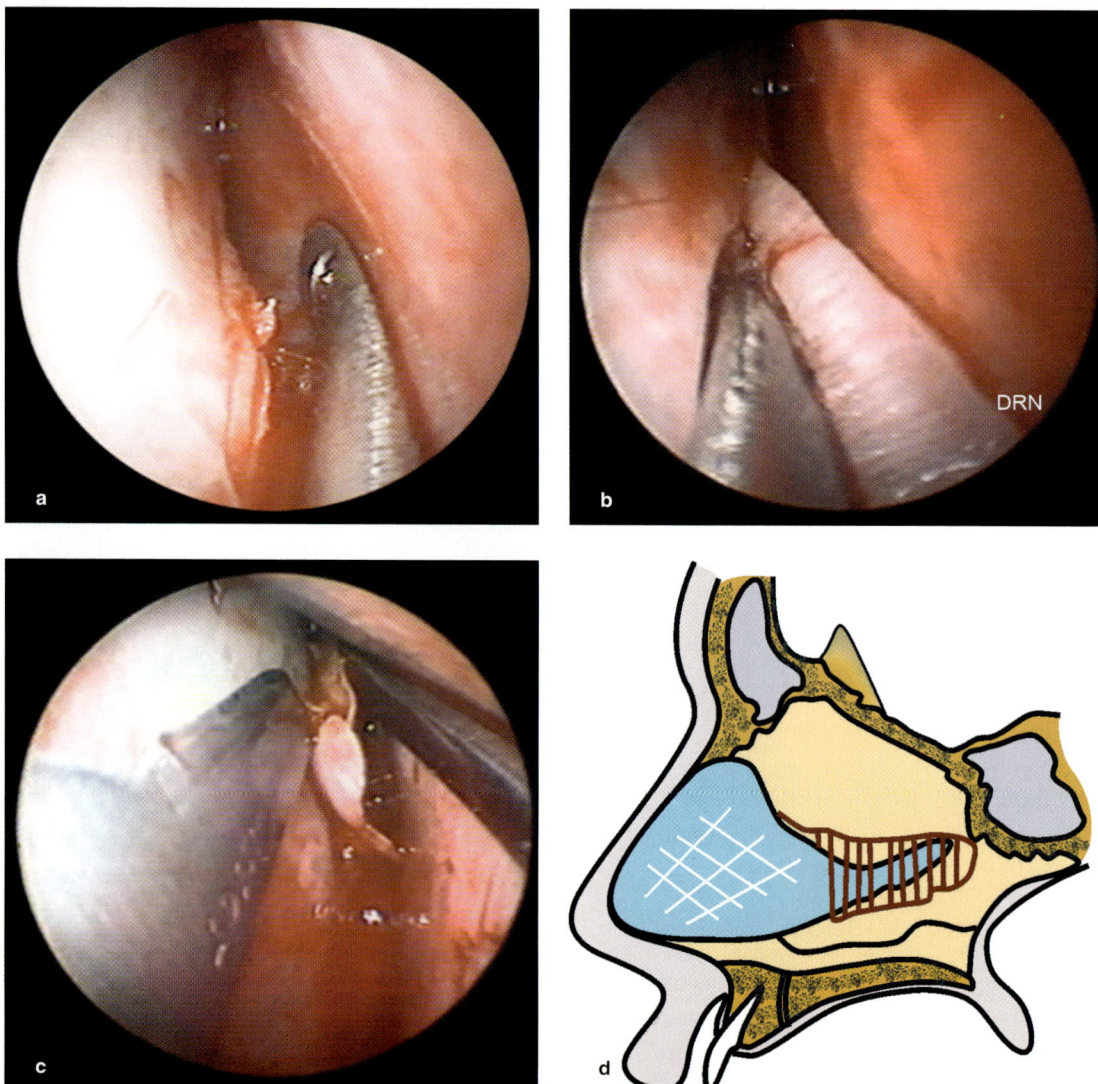

**Fig. 13.1:** **a.** Video endoscopic photograph showing elevation of the mucoperichondrial flap, **b.** Resection of excess cartilage of the maxillary crest, **c.** Shaving of thickened cartilage from vomero-chondral and ethmoido-chondral junction and resection of the thick portion of the vomer and inferior part of the perpendicular plate of ethmoid, **d.** Showing the area of the cartilage and bone resection and criss-cross incision on the concave side of the cartilage

13. **Turbinoplasty** (Fig. 13.3): Inferior turbinate: Inferolateral excision of the inferior turbinate, trimming of the paradoxically turned turbinates, resection of the mulberry hypertrophy of the turbinate by amputation of the posterior end. Middle turbinate: Posterolateral resection for hypertrophied turbinates or lateral partial resection in case of concha bullosa (Nayak *et al.* 2001 and 2002).

14. Splinting is done after a stab incision is made in the inferior aspect of the muco-periosteal flap close to the floor on one side before the closure of the flap, to

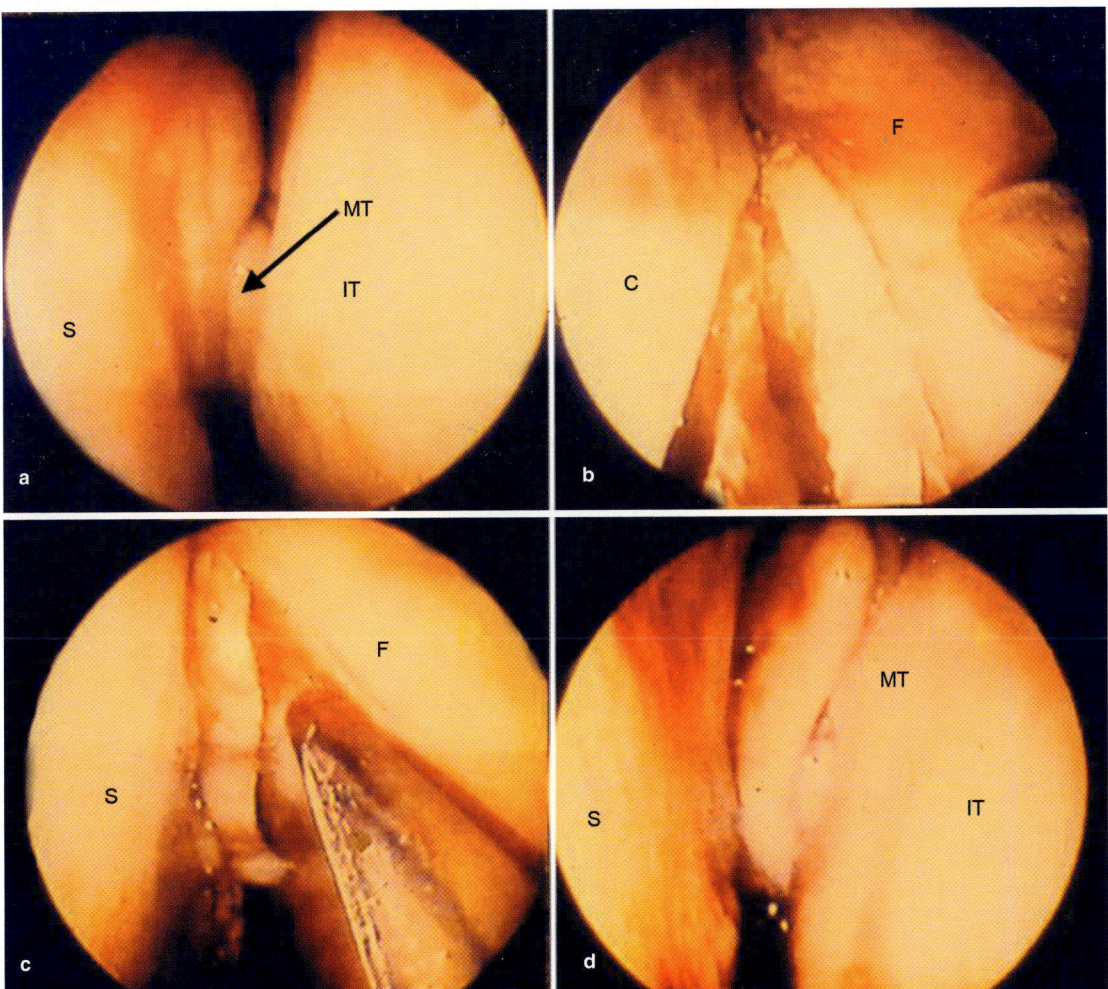

**Fig. 13.2:** The steps of endoscopic septoplasty. **a.** Gross posterior deviation with septo-turbinal compression and subluxation of septal cartilage over maxillary crest, **b.** Resection of subluxated cartilage from the crest, **c.** Shaving of thickened cartilage from vomero-ethmoido-chondral junction with 15 blade Bard-Parker knife, **d.** After correction

prevent hematoma formation. The splinting is done by using prefashioned dental wax plate (baseplate wax) sterilized in Cidex solution and anchored by catgut sutures (Nayak *et al*. 1995) and can be kept for longer period, if synechiae formation is anticipated after endoscopic sinus surgery, in which case an additional wax plate is kept between middle turbinate and lateral wall.

The advantages of nasal endoscope in septal surgery (Nayak *et al*. 1998):

1. Facilitates accurate identification pathology and improved accessibility to remote areas.
2. Better understanding of the lateral wall pathology associated with the septal deformity.
3. Allows limited incision and elevation of the flaps without compromising adequate exposure of the pathological site.

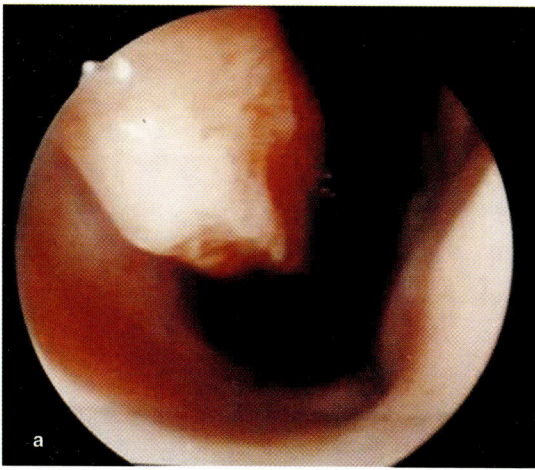 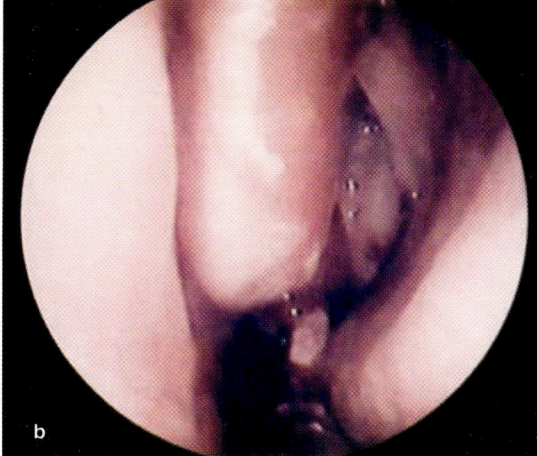

**Fig. 13.3:** The inferior lateral partial resection (turbinoplasty) of **a.** inferior turbinate, **b.** middle turbinate

4. Allows correct identification of the cleavage planes of flap elevation especially in revision and difficult post-traumatic cases.

5. Elevation of flaps in the correct plane minimizes intra-operative bleeding. Moreover, troublesome bleeding due to removal of bony spurs and from remote areas can be managed better with bipolar cautery using endoscopic aid.

6. Allows realignment by limited and precise resection of the pathological areas and/or by precise repair, by strategically placed wedge resections/shaving of cartilage.

7. Unlike the nasal speculum, the endoscope does not distort the septal framework during its use.

8. Effectively relieve the contact areas and thus contact headaches by allowing accurate intraoperative assessment (Nayak-Balakrishna 2012).

9. Allows ultra conservative as well as effective septal surgery thus not jeopardizing the development of the nose and the mid-face in children. Ultra-conservation also preserves the support of external framework, thus allowing better concomitant rhinoplasty.

10. With landmarks well preserved, it keeps the option open for revision surgery, if indicated.

11. Helps in accurate nasal splinting thus avoiding the morbidities of nasal packing.

12. Simultaneous sinus surgery can be done without the fear of lateralization of middle turbinate and consequent synechiae formation.

13. Helps in teaching septal anatomy, pathology and surgery.

14. Helps in documentation

The limitations of the nasal endoscope use may include loss of binocular vision, need for frequent cleaning of the tip of the endoscope especially when there is more bleeding and that combined traditional and endoscopic methods may be required if pathology also involves the caudal most part of the septum, i.e. anterior buckling and trimming of excess caudal end of the septum.

Endoscopic septo-turbinoplasty for a deviated nasal septum is a viable alternative to conventional septal surgery. This is safe, effective and conservative with future scope for revision surgery. The author advocates combination of approaches—endoscopic for the inaccessible middle and posterior part and traditional to accessible anterior most portion of the nasal septum.

## REFERENCES AND FURTHER READING

1. Cottle MH et al. Archives of Otolaryngology, 1958; 68: 301.

2. Freer.O. Journal of American Medical Association, 1902; 38: 636.

3. Killian G. Archiv fur Laryngologie and Rhinologie, 1904; 16: 362

4. Maran AGD. Journal of Laryngology and Otology, 1974; 88: 393–402.

5. Metzenbaum M. Archives of Otolaryngology 1929 9: 282.

6. Nayak DR et al. Journal of Postgraduate Medicine, 1995; 41: 70–1.

7. Nayak DR et al. Journal of Laryngology and Otology, 1998; 112: 934–39.

8. Nayak DR et al. ENT Journal, 2001; Vol. 80, No. 6; 392–403.

9. Nayak DR et al. Indian Journal of Otolaryngology and Head and Neck Surgery, 2002; 54, No. 1: 20–22 Jan–Mar.

10. Nayak DR and Balakrishna R. Indian Journal of Otolaryngol and Head and Neck Surgery; 2012; 64(2):167–171.

11. Galloway T. Plastic repair of the deflected nasal septum arch. Otolaryngology 1946;44:141.

12. Giles et al. Endoscopic septoplasty. Laryngoscope 1994; 104:1507–1509.

13. Murakami WT, Wong LW, Davidso TM. Application of biomechanical behaviour of the cartilage in nasal septoplastic surgery. Laryngoscope (1982); 92,300–309.

# 14

# Endoscopic Dacryocystorhinostomy

Obstruction of the lacrimal system, either congenital or acquired is a common problem. There are multiple causes of the nasolacrimal duct obstruction, the most common of which is recurrent dacryocystitis. The contributing factors include nasal allergy, septal deviation and sinusitis. The nasolacrimal duct obstruction can be corrected with dacryocystorhinostomy (DCR) by creating a fistula between lacrimal sac and nasal cavity. The most common indication for DCR is stenosis of nasolacrimal duct causing annoying epiphora or repeated infection. External DCR was first introduced by Toti in 1904 and transnasal procedure was described by Caldwell in 1893 which was subsequently modified by West in 1911. The transnasal approach did not become popular because of the relative inaccessibility and poor visibility and problem of bleeding during surgery.

These limitations are overcome by the use of nasal endoscope for dacryocystorhino stomy, as popularized by McDonough and Meiring 1989. Endoscopic endonasal dacryocystorhinostomy (EDCR) is considered to be superior alternative technique to conventional external DCR and is quite successful in failed cases of external DCR.

## Tests to Find Nasolacrimal Obstruction

• The Jones test is a test of the patency of the nasolacrimal system. The test is performed by placing fluorescein in the conjunctival sac and seeing whether or not this fluorescein can be visualized in the nose. If after a period of five minutes there is impaired outflow, it is likely that there is an obstruction somewhere in the duct or somewhere in the system. If dye is not seen in the nose after five minutes, then a secondary test can be performed by irrigating the duct. If after irrigating the duct no dye is found in the nose, the dye has never really reached the lacrimal sac to begin with. The obstruction is likely proximal. If dye is seen in irrigate, then dye did reach the nasolacrimal sac, and it is likely that the obstruction is distal.

• Dacryocystogram
• Dacryoscintigraphy with radio labelled materials
• CT scan

## Operative Technique of Endoscopic DCR

This surgery can be done both under local or general anesthesia. The local anesthetic technique is similar to that described under the chapter endoscopic sinus surgery. Topical 2% xylocaine should also be instilled into the conjunctival sac. The lateral wall anterior to the attachment of the middle turbinate was infiltrated submucosally with 2% xylocaine with 1 in 2 lakh dilution of adrenaline using 0 to 30° nasal endoscopic in all the cases (including cases under GA). A, U, C shaped mucoperiosteal flap is created in the lateral wall which is superiorly or posteriorly based 1 square cm size anterior to the attachment of middle turbinate to expose the lacrimal bones or 1 square cm of raw area can be created over

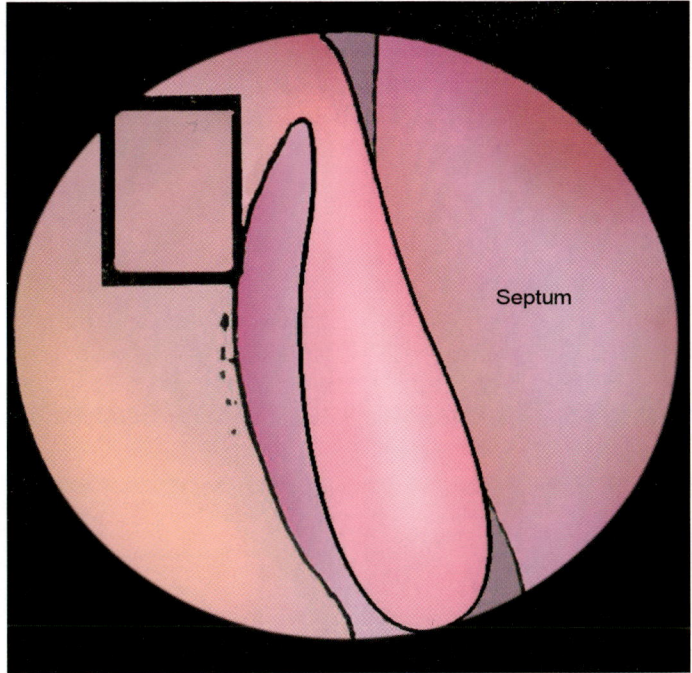

**Fig. 14.1:** The black square area just another to the attachment of middle turbinate (MT) where a raw area has to be created to expose the bone

the lateral wall at the same site by using diathermy/bipolar cautery or laser (shown as black square area in Fig. 14.1).

The lacrimal bone thus exposed was drilled initially using a cutting burr and later a diamond burr to expose the sac. The sac can easily be identified from the surrounding periostium. At this stage saline infiltration can be done through the lacrimal punctum, which will allow the sac to expand and thus can be identified easily (Fig. 14.2).

The bone can also be removed by using a Kerrison rongeur after initial exposure with a drill chisel or gauge should be avoided to prevent penetrating of small bony spicule into the soft tissue and can cause secondary infection and closure of fistula site. After the complete exposure of the sac, the trained assisting surgeon or ophthalmologist is asked to pass a lacrimal probe. The lacrimal sac can also be inflated with normal saline by using syringe for irrigation of lacrimal sac. Irrigation

is important if KTP laser is to be used to prevent damage to the mucosa within the sac. KTP-532 laser is applied over the exposed and inflated sac, till free flow of saline comes out through the fistula thus created (Fig. 14.3).

The sac can also be opened by tenting the lacrimal sac as described above and opening it with a sickle knife. A portion of the medial sac mucosa should be everted, to prevent closure (Figs 14.2a to h). No stenting with silastic tube is required. However, for revision DCR silastic tube stenting is required after creation of the opening in the lacrimal sac.

A jelco cannula no. 20 is used along with the lacrimal probe like a trocar. Once jelco is inserted into the nasal cavity through the lower punctum, the lacrimal probe is removed keeping the cannula in place. Then a silastic cannula of appropriate size is passed through the jelco and brought out through the nasal cavity. Keeping it *in situ*, the jelco cannula is removed. The silastic cannula can be removed after 3–6 weeks.

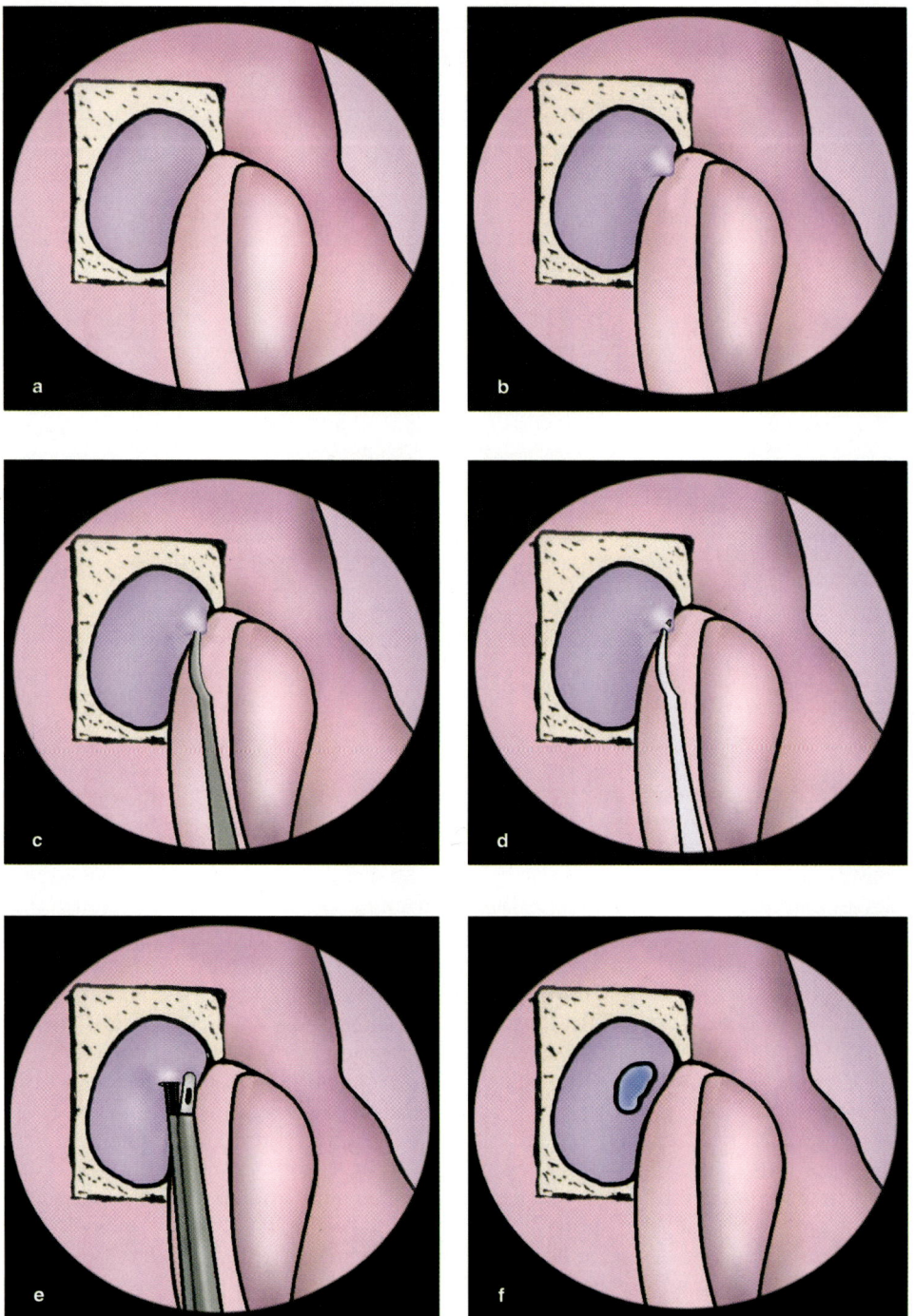

**Fig. 14.2:** Steps of endoscopic dacryocystorhinostomy. **a.** Exposure of the sac, **b.** Tenting of the sac by passing a lacrimal probe through lower punctum into the sac, **c** and **d.** Opening of the sac with sickle knife, **e.** Enlargement of the opening in the sac with the help of through cutting forceps, **f.** Completion of dacryocystorhinostomy

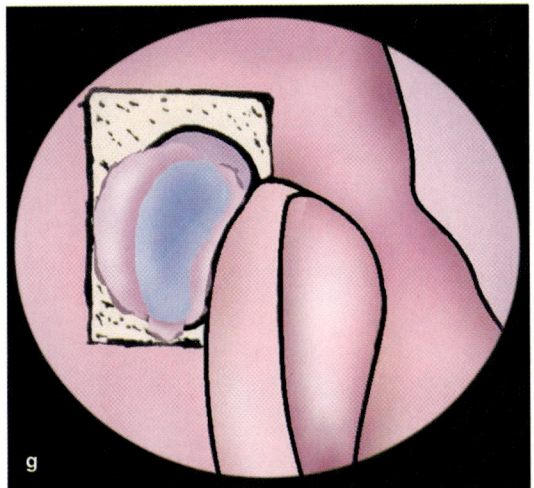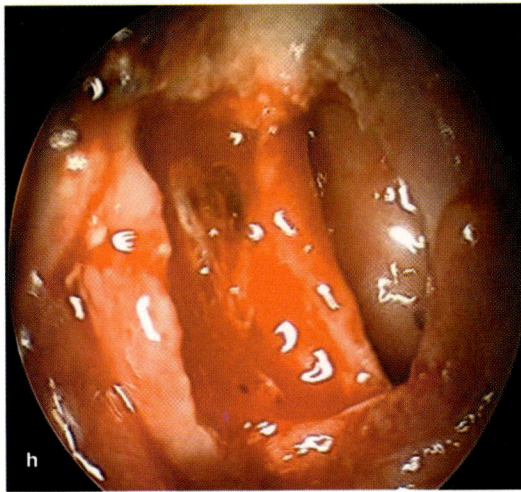

**Fig. 14.2:** Steps of endoscopic dacryocystorhinostomy. **g.** The mucosal flap is everted and reflected into the nasal cavity to complete the endoscopic dacryocystorhinostomy. This prevents closure of rhinostomy site, **h.** Endoscopic picture showing sac being opened and the mucosal margin has been everted

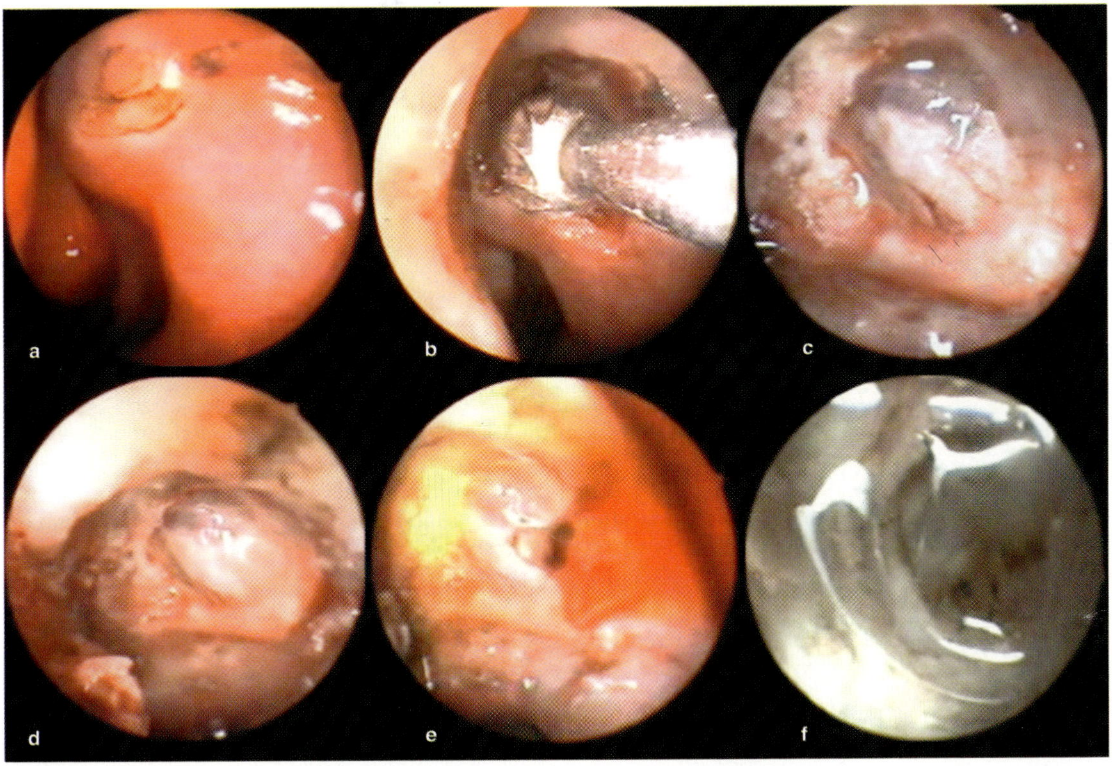

**Fig. 14.3:** **a.** Mucosa is vaporized with KTP532 laser to expose the lacrimal bone, **b.** Lacrimal bone is drilled to expose the sac, **c.** Lacrimal sac is exposed, **d.** Sac is inflated with saline, **e.** Inflated sac is opened with KTP532 laser, **f.** Free flow of saline is noted after creation of an adequate size opening in the sac

## Postoperative Care

1. The nasal cavity should be cleaned
2. Granulation tissue if any should be removed and cauterized. Silastic cannula is one of the causes for granulation, and should be removed immediately if granulation appears. The nose should be irrigated in every alternate day for a period of 7–10 days.
3. Irrigation should be started from the 1st postoperative day in case of primary DCR without cannulation and should be continued weekly intervals till the healing is complete (Fig. 14.4).

### Causes for Failure

The most common cause of a surgical failure in endoscopic DCR is obstruction of the neo-ostium by granulation tissue or synechia that forms post-operatively. Inadequate exposure of the lacrimal sac, due to limited resection of bone and excessive and unnecessary removal or injury of surrounding nasal and lacrimal sac mucosa, and, hence, exposure of bone around a small neo-ostium, appear to contribute to obstruction of the neo-ostium by granulation tissue (Jin, et al. 2006). DNS should be corrected prior to endoscopic DCR. Sinusitis should be treated with functional endoscopic sinus surgery. Silastic cannulation

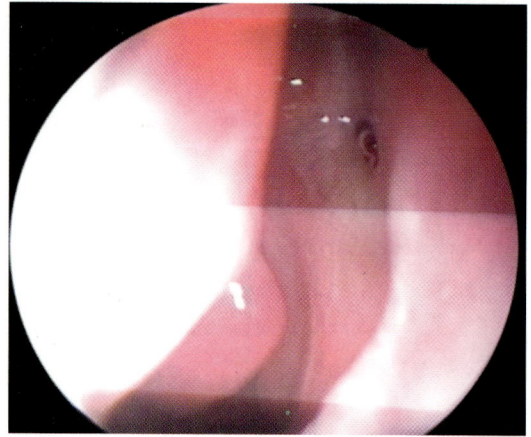

**Fig. 14.4:** Postoperative endoscopic DCR site which is well epithelialized and healed with patent DCR opening

if used should not be kept for a longer period as it can produce granulation and subsequent closure after tube is removed.

### Complications

- Hemorrhage during surgery
- CSF rhinorrhea due to fracture of the ethmoid
- Corneal injury
- Orbital cellulitis
- Granulations
- Synechia
- Lacrimal sump syndrome and reinfection

## REFERENCES AND FURTHER READING

1. Nayak DR, Hazarika P, Rodrigues R AW, Pillai S, Balakrishnan R. Endoscopic dacryocystorhinostomy vs KTP 532 laser-assisted endoscopic dacryocystorhinostomy; Indian Journal of Otolaryngology and Head and Neck Surgery, 2005; 57 (4), 278–282.
2. Nayak DR, Satish R, Shah Parul, Poojary K and Balakrishnan R. Endoscopic dacryocystorhinostomy and retrograde nasolacrimal duct dilatation with cannulation-our experience. Indian Journal of Otolaryngology and Head and Neck Surgery 1999–2000: 52(1): 23–27, ISSN 0019–5421.
3. Rice DN. Endoscopic dacryocystorhinostomy: a cadaveric study. Ann of rhinol, 1998; 2,127–128.
4. Toti A. Nuovo metodo conservatore di eura radicale delle suporazioni chroniche del sacco lacrimale (dacriocistorhinostomia). Clin Mod Firenze 1904;10:385–9.
5. Caldwell. Two new operation for obstruction of the nasal duct. New York Medical Journal 1893;57:581–2.
6. Weston JM. A window resection of nasal duct in case of stenosis. Transaction of Am. Oph Society 1910;12(Pt2) 654–8.
7. McDonough M, Meiring JH. Endoscopic transnasal DCR, JLO 1989;103(6):585–7.
8. Jin HR, et al. Endoscopic Dacryocystorhinostomy: Creation of a Large Marsupialized Lacrimal Sac; J Korean Med Sci. 2006 August; 21(4):719–723.

# 15

# Management of Nasal Allergy

Nasal allergy is a very common condition and it frequently acts as a triggering factor for both acute and chronic rhinosinusitis. Nasal inflammation associated with allergic rhinitis can cause obstruction in the area of osteo-meatal complex, thereby predisposing to bacterial infection of the sinuses. This process accounts for many cases of acute and chronic bacterial sinusitis. The term allergic rhino-sinusitis is the most appropriate terminology when nasal allergy is associated with sinusitis. Patients with perennial allergic rhinitis—especially those with significant sensitivity to moulds and/or house dust mites—are parti-cularly susceptible to acute sinusitis and many patients with chronic sinusitis also have nasal allergy. Thus, failing in the management of nasal allergy can lead to treatment failure in sinusitis. Therefore it is essential to include nasal allergy management in the treatment strategy for chronic sinusitis.

## ALLERGIC RHINITIS

### History

- First described by John Bostock in 1819 as seasonal catarrah
- 1873, Blackley observed the first reaction by applying pollen to excoriated skin
- 1911, treatment began by Leonard Noon on the assumption of antitoxins.

### Definition

It is an acute IgE mediated, type-1 hyper-sensitivity reaction of nasal mucosa in response to antigenic substance [allergen] associated with episodic attacks of sneezing, watery rhinorrhea, watering of the eyes. Patient may also present with tightness of chest due to subclinical bronchospasm.

### Types

- Seasonal (or intermittent) allergic rhinitis (most often referred to as hay fever) is triggered by air borne pollen most comm-only from grasses, weeds and sometimes trees.
- Perennial (or persistent) allergic rhinitis occurs throughout the year and is most commonly triggered by exposure to house dust mites.
- Mixed when both seasonal and perennial type coexist.

Allergic rhinitis is a chronic disease where causation is multifactorial and manifestation is multifocal. It is very important to obtain a proper history with respect to various predisposing factors and possible causative agent (allergen), the pathophysiological mechanism and progress of nasal allergy. The symptom of patient and the type of allergy depends on a number of factors.

### Precipitating Factors

#### Aerobiological Flora

This is determined by the allergens present in that environment of which inhalant allergen is more common.

## Common Allergens

I. Inhalant: Commonest cause
  - Pollen and dust including house dust mite—75%
  - Fungus
  - Animal danders
  - Miscellaneous.

  House dust mite species are the most common type of allergen present in house dust that is associated with allergic rhinitis. These mites feed on organic material in households, particularly the skin that is shed from humans and pets. They can be found in carpets, upholstered furniture, pillows, mattresses, comforters, and stuffed toys. While they thrive in warmer temperatures and high humidity, they can be found year-round in many households. On the other hand, dust mites are rare in arid climates.

II. Food allergy

## Predisposing Factors

a. *Age:* Patients with any age are susceptible to allergy. However, young patients are more affected. About 70% of the cases present with symptoms of nasal allergy before 30 years of age (Yadav *et al*. 2003).

b. *Sex:* Males are more commonly affected with male to female ratio of about 3:2. Some report equal predilection.

c. *Industrialization and urbanization:* Incidence of allergic rhinitis is ever increasing because of industrialization and urbanization responsible for environment pollution. Reported incidence of allergic rhinitis is 1.4–39. 7% of population in the western countries. In UK there is four-fold increase in incidence of allergic rhinitis in last thirty years.

d. Genetic predisposition plays a significant role in allergic manifestation. Chances of getting allergic rhinitis are more if one or more parents are suffering from allergy.

e. Focal sensitivity of nasal mucosa can trigger the allergic reaction.

f. IgA deficiency state makes the patient more prone for allergy.

g. Psychology

h. *Living conditions:* Residential and workplace conditions play a significant role in the etiology. Crowding, dusty environment, air-conditioned rooms may predispose. Dust may accumulate in the carpets, curtains, bed sheets, bookshelves, store shelves, etc. and its exposure may precipitate the allergic response in genetically predisposed individuals. Allergy may be an occupational hazard also wherein the individual is exposed to allergen in his workplace. Example: Librarian, storekeeper, factory worker, etc.

i. *Environment:* Depends on the aerobiological flora of the particular environment. Climatic conditions including season, altitude can affect the manifestation of the symptoms. Based on this the allergic manifestations may be classified into seasonal and perennial allergic rhinitis. In seasonal allergic rhinitis, the symptoms are more in a particular season. Example: Pollens in spring, fungus in rainy season, etc. In perennial the symptoms are present throughout the year. Common examples are house dust mite, pets, etc. (Fig. 15.1).

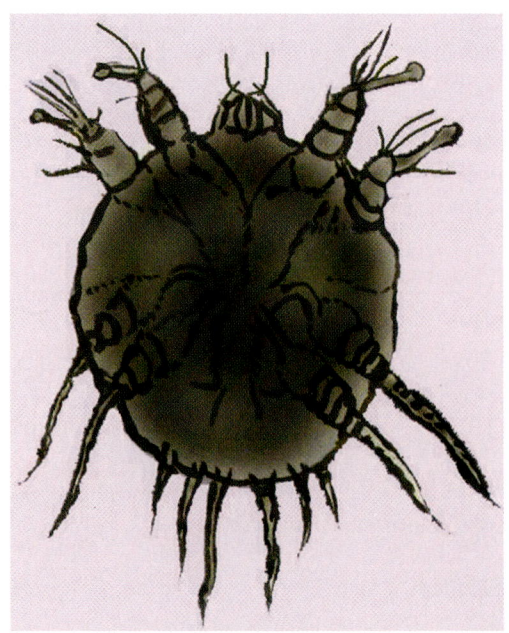

**Fig. 15.1:** House dust mite

## Pathophysiology

### *Primary Response*

This is also called priming. After initial exposure to the allergen (antigen), in genetically predisposed individual, specific antibody is produced which gets fixed to the mast cells and basophils. This sensitizes the nasal mucosa to this allergen. Allergic challenge occurs in less than 24 hr and the reversal starts 48 hr after. It is mainly mediated by histamine.

### *Local Phenomenon*

It occurs in response to the chemical mediators leading to mucosal edema associated with sneezing and rhinorrhea.

### *Non-specific Response*

It occurs due to non-specific stimuli like pollutants, salicylates, cold weather, air-conditioning, etc. This can initiate a response similar to priming and can precipitate symptoms.

## Mechanism (Fig. 15.2)

### *Clinical Features*

#### *Symptoms*

The symptoms may be seasonal or perennial. All symptoms are simply a manifestation of the body's defense mechanism to the allergen.

#### *Classical*

Mainly seen in seasonal allergic rhinitis. This includes paroxysmal bouts of sneezing, watery rhinorrhea and nasal obstruction with itching of the nose on exposure to known or unknown allergen. This may be associated with non-nasal manifestations like watering and itching of the eyes, itching of the palate and skin and in some it may be associated

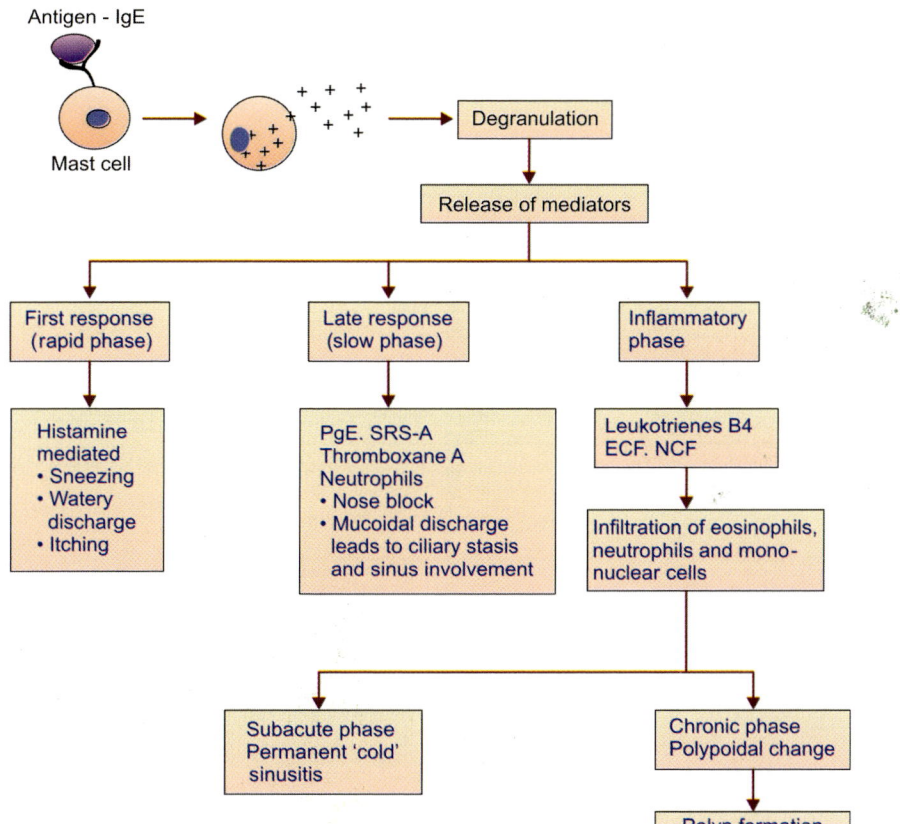

**Fig. 15.2:** Mechanism of allergic rhinitis

with bronchospasm, which may be sub-clinical. Patient may complain of hyposmia or anosmia depending on the severity of the disease.

In perennial allergy the symptoms are usually less severe and may present as recurrent cold or nasal stuffiness with sneezing and watery rhinorrhea.

### Signs

- Pale bluish edematous nasal mucosa (Fig. 15.3)
- Bulky edematous turbinates with bluish/purplish tinge of the mucosa
- Mucosa coated with clear/mucoid secretions
- In advanced cases the mucosa of the middle turbinate may be polypoidal and frank polyposis may be seen in the middle meatus (Fig. 15.4).
- Septum may be thickened due to mucosal swelling.

### Classical signs associated with allergic rhinitis

- Overriding maxillary incisors
- High arched palate

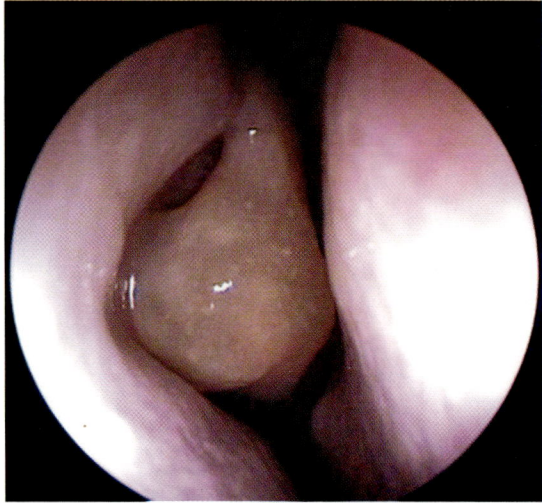

**Fig. 15.4:** Polypoidal changes of middle turbinate

- Allergic shiners (Fig. 15.5)
- Allergic salute
- Transverse crease above the tip of nose and lower eyelids (Fig. 15.6).
- Conjunctival congestion
- Periorbital swelling.

### Diagnosis

Patient with the following features should be considered allergic rhinitis.
- Recurrent upper respiratory infections
- Frequent sore throats
- Mouth breathing and snoring
- A feeling of pressure over the sinuses
- Recurrent infective sinusitis

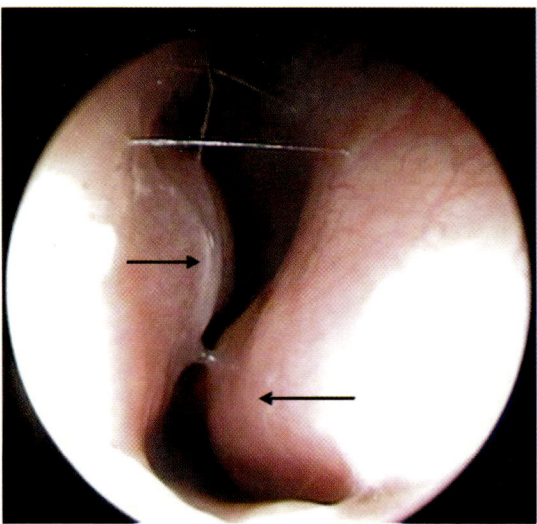

**Fig. 15.3:** Endoscopic picture showing the pale edematous turbinates with septal spur coated with clear mucoid secretions [Turbinate (→), septal spur (←)]

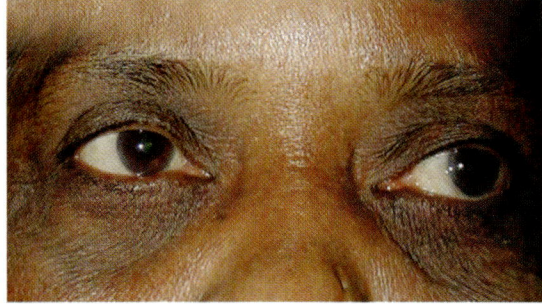

**Fig. 15.5:** Dark circle around the eyes (allergic shiners)

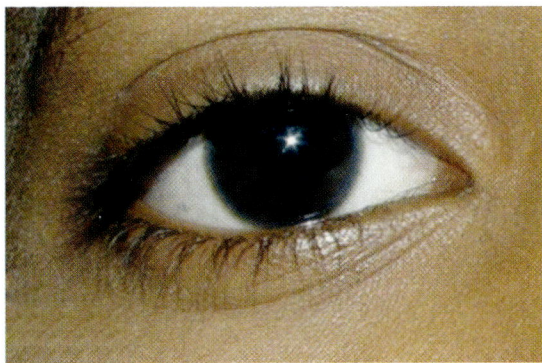

**Fig. 15.6:** Transverse crease below the lower eyelid

- Headaches
- Recurrent upper respiratory tract or middle ear infections, particularly in children.

### Differential Diagnosis

1. Common cold
2. Vasomotor rhinitis
3. Chronic sinusitis
4. Rhinitis medicamentosa
5. Occupational rhinitis

### Investigations

*Non-specific*

Nasal smear for eosinophils
- Total WBC count and differential count
- Absolute eosinophil count
- Histamine test

**Specific** *(Qualitative and quantitative tests)*

**1. In vivo tests**
- *Skin tests*
  i. *Subcuticular test—Prick/scratch test:* This is the most popular, practical and safe test. It may be used as a screening test. Prick test is more preferred. This test is more readily reproducible, has lower incidence of false positive results, is more accurate and has less risk of anaphylaxis. In this test, a drop of test extract solution (allergen with histamine and saline as control) is placed on the unprepared skin of the medial aspect of

forearm. Using a lancet at about 45 degrees to the skin through the drop, the epidermis is pricked with a lifting motion. Care is taken not to penetrate the dermis. The area is examined after 10 minutes for histamine control and after 20 minutes for the allergen. Wheal response around the prick is measured and compared with standardized scales. In India, Shivapuri criteria are used to quantify the severity of the wheal response. Anafilatic reaction can occur while doing allergic test and it is necessary to have the emergency kit while doing allergy test (Fig. 15.7). Prick test is contraindicated in cases with dermographism, patients with antihistaminic, anti-inflammatory or decongestant treatment (Fig. 15.8).

ii. *Intradermal skin test:* This has higher chances of anaphylaxis and has to be done only with resuscitation drugs and equipment ready.

iii. *Skin end-point titration test:* This is a quantitative intradermal skin test for specific allergen. This test is done using a dilute and known concentration of an allergen, which is injected intradermally, and the response is noted. The dose is increased gradually intradermal skin test technique using 1:5 serial dilutions of allergenic extract. This technique is safe, reliable and is well standardized intradermal injec-

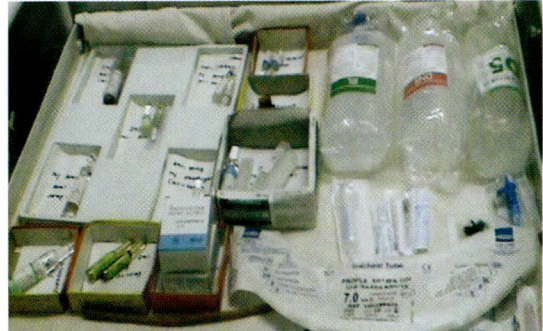

**Fig. 15.7:** Emergency kit consisting of injectable antihistamines like avil, Inj. adrenaline, endotracheal tube, saline infusion, etc.

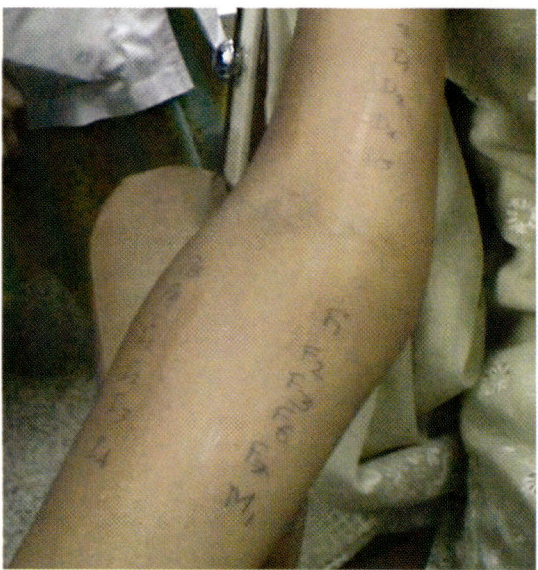

**Fig. 15.8:** Prick test

tions of 0.01 ml allergenic extract applied to the upper lateral arm. Wheal and Flare beyond 5 mm suggest positive response. Maximal whealing occurs at 15 minutes. The endpoint is defined as the antigen dilution which yields a wheal at least 2 mm larger than the preceding negative wheal, and which is followed by a wheal at the next stronger dilution. The confirming wheal is important for determining the true endpoint.

iv. *Nasal challenge (nasal provocation) test:* Not a very popular test due to potential risks of anaphylaxis and has limited clinical applications. The test dose is delivered in a nebulizer using a specific allergen.

v. *Nasal cytology:* It can be done using a dry wipe technique without surface anesthesia. The specimen is applied to the slide with a firm rolling action. The smear is fixed immediately with 95% alcohol and is stained with Wright-Giemsa stain. Following cell types are noted.

- Eosinophils
- Mast cells/basophils/both

- Epithelial cells
- Lymphocytes
- Neutrophils
- Goblet cells

In allergy patients have increased eosinophils of more than 10%.

**2. In vitro tests**

i. *Radio-allergo-sorbant test (RAST):* This is very useful test especially in case with dermographism. This is less sensitive than skin prick test but is more expensive. RAST allows measurement of the amount of specific IgE to individual allergens in a sample of blood. The amount of specific IgE produced to a particular allergen approximately correlates with the allergic sensitivity to that substance. These tests allow determination of specific IgE to a number of different allergens from one blood sample, but the sensitivity and specificity are not always as good as accurate skin testing (depending on the laboratory and assay used for the RAST). As with skin testing, virtually all of the allergens that cause allergic rhinitis can be determined using the RAST, although testing for some allergens is less well established compared to others.

ii. *Fluoro-allergo-sorbent test (FAST):* The fluoro-allergo-sorbent test (FAST) is similar to the ELISA, except for the use of a fluorogenic substrate which produces fluorescence that can be read with a fluorometer. The test procedure can be completed in 6 hours. There is good correlation with skin prick test and RAST against aero-allergens. An automatel version of the FAST, the CAP system is now available. It is claimed that its sensitivity and specificity are better than RAST. Being automated, it has a faster turnaround time and is less demanding on human resources. Results are expressed in kilo units per liter which is advantageous for comparison with other techniques.

iii. *MAST CLA:* The multiple allergosorbent test chemiluminescent assays (MAST

CLA) have shown good correlation with skin prick test and RAST against several aero-allergens. In this assay, allergens are coated onto threads. It performs simultaneous determination of total IgE and 35 allergen specific IgE in serum.

iv. Paper immunoallegrosorbant test (PRIST) is a recognized effective test for the determination of serum concentration of IgE antibody.

### Other tests

These are done to rule out associated sinus pathology and polyposis.
a. X-ray PNS
b. CT OMC
c. Diagnostic nasal endoscopy

## TREATMENT OF ALLERGIC RHINITIS

### Therapeutic Goals

These include medical line of management with short, medium and long-term goals.

1. Short-term relief that usually helps within days (medication).
2. Medium-term measures to reduce reliance on medication (allergen avoidance, if possible).
3. Long-term options including immunotherapy, particularly if medication is poorly tolerated or ineffective and allergen avoidance is difficult.

### Medical

#### 1. Pharmacotherapy

a. *Antihistamines:* This is the mainstay of treatment for allergic rhinitis, when avoidance of allergens is not possible. It is most preferred during the acute attack. These are basically H-1 receptor antagonists and block the effect of histamine on the receptors. Various antihistamines are available and the recent ones like fexofenadine, loratidine, rupatidine levocetrizine, etc., have faster onset of action, longer duration and with less side effects like sedation and cardiovascular changes and anti-cholinergic effects. Antihistamine

nasal sprays and eye drop—antihistamines like azelastine (Azep) can be used as a nasal spray with no long term side effects. It acts rapidly (within minutes) to relieve sneezing or itching and are generally well tolerated. In general, they are less effective at relieving severe nasal congestion.

TAK-427 is a long-acting antihistamine under trial, which suppresses acute phase of allergic reactions and may have a long-lasting antihistamine activity with minimum sedative side effect.

b. *Steroids:* They act by inhibiting the inflammatory reaction. Systemic steroids can be given in short course in seasonal or perennial allergic rhinitis. Steroid nasal sprays like beclomethasone, budesonide, fluticasone, mometasone, etc. are particularly useful as they have lesser side-effects and may be used for longer period. Reduction in middle meatal edema may facilitate drainage of the sinus secretions. Long-term use may cause crusting and fungal colonization.

c. *Anticholinergic sprays:* Ipratopium bromide nasal spray is very effective in reducing watery rhinorrhoea.

d. *Sodium chromoglycate:* Mast cell stabilizing nasal sprays or eye drops (e.g. Ifiral/Fintal) reduce inflammation by stabilizing the mast cells and preventing its degranulation. It is available as nasal drops or nasal spray for allergic rhinitis/eye drops for allergic conjunctivitis. This is mainly used for prophylaxis and therefore should be used regularly and before the attack.

e. *Decongestants:* They are useful to reduce nasal obstruction and mucosal edema and rhinorrhea. Oral preparations are available with antihistamines. Long-term use of topical decongestants is best avoided as they can cause rhinitis medicamentosa and should not be given for more than 4–5 days. Oral preparations include pseudo-ephedrine hydrochloride, phenyphefrine hydrochloride, etc. Topical decongestants include oxymetazoline, xylometazoline, ephedrine in saline, etc.

f. *Saline irrigation of the nasal cavities:* Help in removing secretions and prevent secondary infection.

g. *Ramatroban:* Nasal obstruction is currently thought to be closely related to the presence and abundance of lipid mediators, such as leukotriene and thromboxane (TX) A2. The novel drug ramatroban, a TXA2 receptor antagonist, has been demonstrated, in clinical trials, to improve nasal obstruction in the treatment of patients with allergic rhinitis and it has recently become commercially available. Ramatroban suppresses the secretion of chemical mediators in nasal mucosa that are thought to be involved in the allergic reaction in patients with perennial allergic rhinitis.

## Avoidance of Allergen

This is ideal but is not always possible. Some of the known allergens can be avoided, like paper dust, house dust, animal dander, etc. by avoiding pets, washing curtains regularly, keeping less articles in the living room, changing bed sheets and pillow covers frequently, use of ironed bed sheets, pillow covers before use, use of mask/nasal filters while cleaning the house, prefer vacuum cleaning or wet mopping to dry mopping, avoidance of carpets, etc. will control most of the aero-allergens effectively. Seasonal and environmental allergen can be avoided to certain extent by knowing and avoiding the aerobiological flora of that particular environment. Allergic skin tests may be useful in identifying the allergens.

## Immunotherapy (Desensitization)

It is the closest thing to a cure for allergic rhinitis. The role of immunotherapy is limited especially in case of multiple allergens. However, people with allergy to limited number of allergens may find it useful. Immunotherapy is often recommended for treatment of allergic rhinitis (and sometimes asthma) when:

- Symptoms are severe
- The cause is difficult to avoid (e.g. grass pollen)
- Medications are unhelpful or cause adverse side effects; and patients need medication most days.

It is effective only in about 40% of cases and involves the administration of gradually increasing amounts of allergic material, usually given to patients by injection over a period of years. These allergen injections alter the way in which the immune system reacts to allergens, by switching off allergy. It is administered by giving sub-cutaneous injections in diluted form at weekly intervals. The dose is gradually increased till the optimal level is achieved. RAST/skin end point titration based immunotherapy is more effective since the quantitative analysis can be done and the patient can receive higher dose without the fear of anaphylaxis. Hence they get an early response. Immunotherapy helps in reducing the specific serum IgE level and a decrease in basophil sensitivity and increase in IgG blocking antibody level which helps in preventing the allergen from reaching the mast cells and thus preventing their degranulation. The proper selection of allergen extracts is important in maintaining an efficient allergy practice. This article discusses pollen extract selection. The selection of tree, grass, and weed pollen extracts depends very much on where the clinician's practice is located (aerobiological flora).

Sublingual immunotherapy is gaining popularity in recent days and has the distinct advantages over subcutaneous immunotherapy. It can be administered safely with less risk of anaphylaxis than subcutaneous immunotherapy. Gut frequently being exposed to numerous foreign proteins on a constant basis. Its immune system is tolerance to nonpathogenic proteins, that forms the basis for this concept.

Allergen extracts given sublingually are primarily taken up by the dendritic cells in the mucosa and are presented to T cells in the draining lymph nodes. Likely mechanisms of action include activation of T regulatory cells and down regulation of mucosal mast cells. Allergenic proteins that reach the small intestine are processed through columnar mucosal cells and are presented to T lymphocytes within Peer's patches. Changes in the humoral responses to allergens are seen with this technique are 'increased allergen specific lgG4' production under the control of IL-10. There is blunting of seasonal increases in allergen specific lgE. The CD8+ T cells are increased and there is a decrease in the CD4:CD8 T cell ratio. In contrast to the sub-cutaneous immunotherapy, the lgG level decreases in sublingual immunotherapy and is safer and comfortable for patient. It can be taken by the patient himself at home after proper advice. The initial administration needs to be supervised as there is possibility of anaphylactic reaction (Bufe *et al*. 2009, de Goot and Bijl, 2009).

Local nasal immunotherapy is an alternative form of mucosal immunotherapy and its ability to reduce rhinitis symptoms and medication usage, as well as to decrease nasal reactivity towards offending allergen has been well established (Meheta and Smith 1975, Motta *et al*. 2000). Nasal immunotherapy with single allergen (aqueous mixed weed) extract administered with cromolyn sodium pre-treatment for 17 to 21 weeks was effective in reducing both nasal and ocular symptoms of weed pollen-induced allergic rhinitis (Gaglani *et al*. 1997).

*Role of omalizumab:* Omalizumab is a molecularly cloned humanized monoclonal antibody inhibiting human IgE. It binds specifically to the region of the IgE molecule that binds to the IgE receptor on the mast cell or basophils. Studies have shown that Omalizumab is effective in the treatment of seasonal allergic rhinitis (Casale, et al. 2001). The anti-inflammatory effects of omalizumab at different sites of allergic inflammation and the clinical benefits of anti-IgE therapy in patients with allergic asthma and allergic rhinitis emphasize the fundamental importance of IgE in allergic inflammation (Holgate & Casale, et al. 2005).

## Surgical Management

Role of surgery is limited to reduction of the size of the turbinate, correction of septal deviation and limited endoscopic sinus surgery if sinuses are involved. The inferior and the middle turbinate are trimmed by inferolateral partial resection using micro-debrider or turbinectomy scissors. Septal deviation should ideally be dealt with limited ultraconservative endoscopic approach. Limited sinus surgery with preservation of uncinate process may reduce postoperative postnasal discharge, which is often seen following traditional Functional endoscopic sinus surgery (FESS) for allergy associated chronic sinusitis (Nayak *et al*. 2001) including polyposis. Antiallergy treatment should continue even after surgical intervention.

## REFERENCES AND FURTHER READING

1. Nayak DR, Balakrishnan R, Hazarika P. Prevention and management of synaechia in pediatric endoscopic sinus surgery using dental wax plates, International Journal of Pediatric Otolaryngology 1998, 46: 171–8.

2. Nayak DR, Balakrishnan R, Murty KD. Functional anatomy of the uncinate process and its role in endoscopic sinus surgery. Indian Journal of Otolaryngology and Head and Neck Surgery 2001; Jan, 53(1): 27–31.

3. Nayak DR, Balakrishnan R, Murty KD. Endoscopic physiologic approach to allergy associated chronic rhinosinusitis: A Preliminary study. ENT Journal 2001 June; 80(6): 392–403.

4. Yadav, A. Verma, J. Singh Study on Nasal Mucous Clearance in Patients of Perennial Allergic Rhinitis; Indian J Allergy Asthma Immunol 2003; 17(2) : 89–91.

5. Dzul AI. Selecting allergenic extracts for inhalant allergy testing and immunotherapy. Otolaryngol Clin North Am. 1998; Feb; 31(1):11–25.

6. Varghese B, Murthy PSN, Rajan R, Nayak DR, Hazarika P, Murty KD and Mathew KJ. (1995) "Nasobronchial relationship: a controversial entity?". Kerala Journal of ENT, 1995; 3(3); 6–12. 18.

7. Crimi E, Brusasco V, Crimi P, Brancatisano M, Bregante A. (1988). The fluoro-allergosorbent test: a comparison with RAST and skin test in respiratory allergy. Ann Allergy; 61: 371–4. 8.

8. Seltzer JM, Georges M, Halpern M, Tasy YG. Correlation of allergy test results obtained by IgE FAST, RAST and prick-puncture method. Ann Allergy, 1989; 1985; 54: 25–30.

9. Scolozzi R, Boccafogh A, Vicentini L, Baraldi A, Bagni B. Correlation of MAST Chemiluminescent assay (CLA) with RAST and skin prick tests for diagnosis of inhalent allergic disease. Ann Allergy; 1998; 62: 193 a–b.

10. Bufe et al. J Allergy Clin Immunology; 2009, 123(1):167.

11. de Groot H, Bijl A. Allergy. 2009; 64(6):963.

12. Meheta SB, Smith JM. Clin Allergy. 1975; 5:279–86.

13. Gaglani B et al. Ann Allergy Asthma Immunol. 1997 Sep; 79(3):259–65.

14. Motta G.; et al. Laryngoscope 2000 Jan; 110(1):132–9.

15. Casale T. Anti-IgE (omalizuman) therapy in seasonal allergic rhinitis. Am J Resp Crit Care Med 2001; 164:1821.

16. Holgate S, Casale T, et al. The antihistaminic effect of Omalizumab confirm the central role in allergic rhinitis, J Allerg Clin Immunology, 2005, March, 115(3):459–65.

17. Fukuda S. et al. Characteristics of the anti-histamine effect of TAK-427, a novel imidazopyridazine derivative. Inflm Res 2003; May;52(5):206–14.

18. Ohkubo K and Gotoh M. Effect of ramatroban, a thromboxane A2 antagonist, in the treatment of perennial allergic rhinitis, Allergology International (2003)52:131–138.

# 16

# Balloon Sinuplasty

Inflammatory disease of the paranasal sinuses is a common problem that affects millions of people. Functional endoscopic sinus surgery is one of the most accepted modality of surgical treatment for patients who have failed to respond to medical therapy. Over the past 20 years, many patients have benefited from endoscopic sinus surgery.[2] The objective of the functional endoscopic surgery(FES), although it is been discussed by some authors, is to increase the ventilation and draining of the paranasal sinuses involved and allow the return of adequate functioning of the muco-ciliary movements of the nasal mucosa. Many of these patients treated surgically respond poorly to extensive endoscopic surgery and could be benefited with less invasive methods, with major preservation of the nasal mucosa.[1,2] Nayak and collaborators proposed the physiological endoscopic approach, with conservation of the nasal mucosa and the uncinate process in the surgical management of patients with chronic rhinosinusitis asso-ciated with allergic symptoms.[1]

Balloon sinuplasty is a new medical procedure which uses a balloon catheter system to dilate ostium of various major paranasal sinuses similar to the technique used in angioplasty instead of instruments such as microdebriders and forceps. It is currently used in the maxillary, frontal and sphenoid sinuses.[3] Balloon sinuplasty technology was developed by Acclarent, Inc., and was brought to the market in 2005, after FDA approval. This procedure involves the dilation of the desired region, which may lead to 16 pressure atmospheres in the balloon, producing local micro fractures that end up remodeling the anatomy, dilates the ostia and allows a PNS normal aeration without, however, the removal of the tissues and damage to the nasal mucosa. This makes the procedure less invasive than a classical functional endoscopic sinus surgery.[3,4] Excellent results were seen on long-term follow up following balloon sinuplasty.[9]

## BALLOON SINUPLASTY TECHNIQUE

Using a sinus guide catheter and an ultra flexible guide wire the targeted sinus is entered (Fig. 16.1). After confirming with C arm/Relieva Luma system, the sinus balloon catheter is advanced over the sinus guide wire (Fig. 16.2). The balloon is placed at the site of obstruction/stenosed ostium. Once the

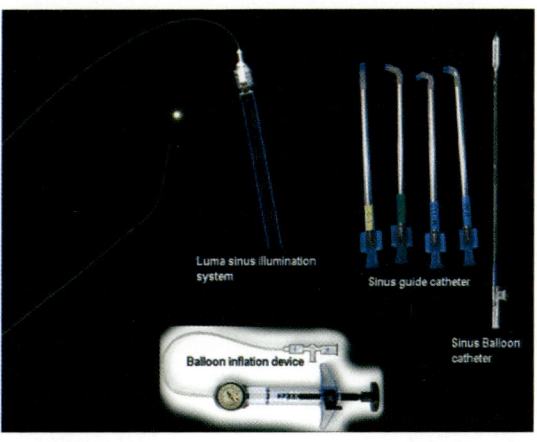

**Fig. 16.1:** Acclarent balloon sinuplasty system

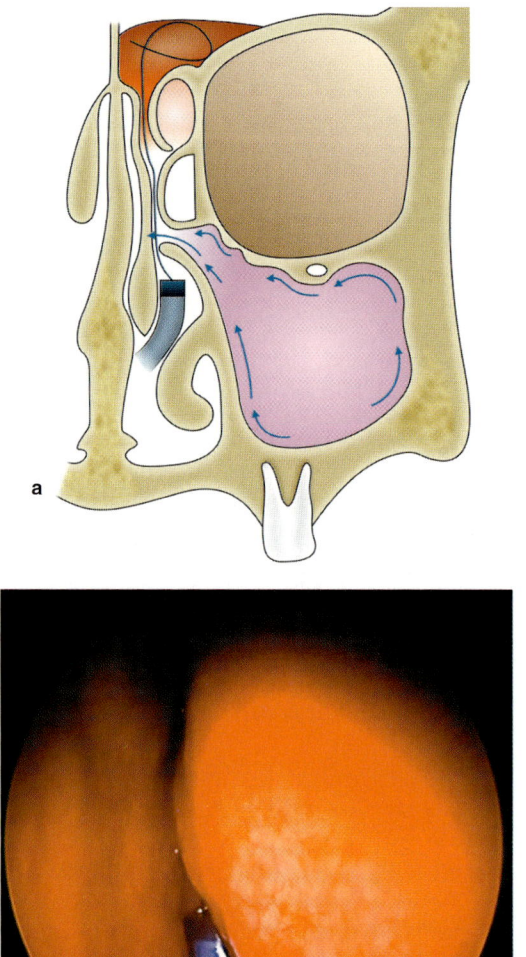

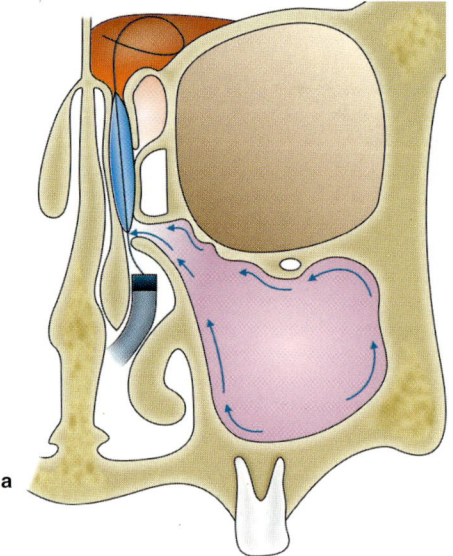

Fig. 16.2: (a) Frontal sinus guide wire being passed into the frontal sinus, (b) after confirmation of guide wire being passed into the frontal sinus by Relieva Luma system, sinus balloon catheter is advanced over the guide wire

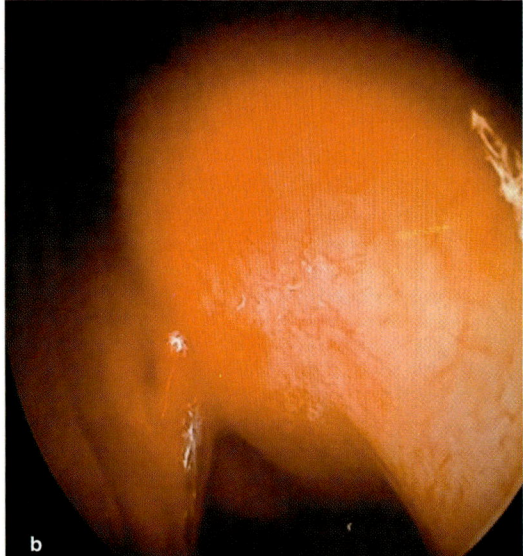

Fig. 16.3: (a) Balloon catheter is dilated after placing at the site of narrow frontal recess and ostium, (b) the inflated balloon after dilatation of the frontal recess

position of the sinus balloon catheter is confirmed, the balloon is gradually inflated with saline (8–10 atmospheres) to open and remodel the narrowed or blocked ostium (Fig. 16.3). The balloon catheter is then deflated and withdrawn (Fig. 16.4) and instead an irrigation catheter is advanced over the guide wire into the affected sinus to irrigate and flush out the tenacious sinus secretions accumulated within. Irrigation catheter is then removed from the targeted sinus (Fig.16.5). The first author of this book (DRN) prefers to place a small elongated piece of nasopore (bio-degradable synthetic polyurethane foam) soaked with povidone iodine solution along with triamcinolone which does

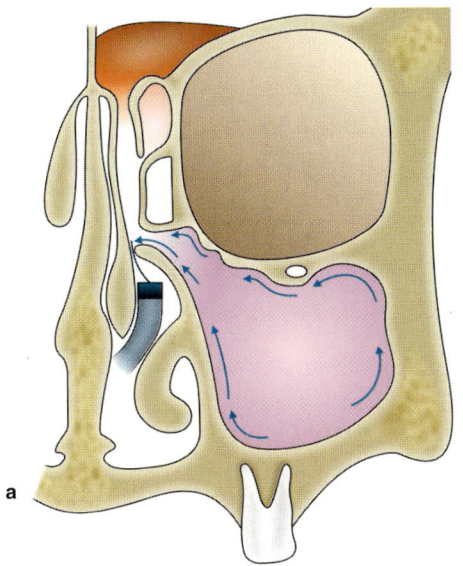

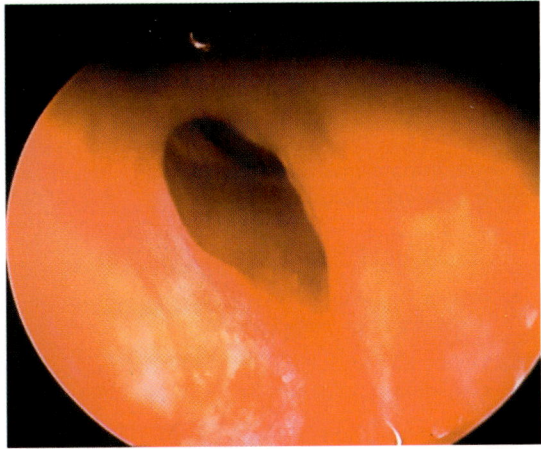

**Fig. 16.5:** The frontal recess and frontal sinus ostium after balloon dilatation

- Early recovery.
- Revision possible.
- Short hospital stay/office based procedure.

### Disadvantages

- Disposable catheter and balloon
- Expensive
- Long-term results have yet to be ascertained
- Not effective in cases of extensive polyposis/allergic fungal sinusitis.

### Complications

The potential complications include CSF leak, orbital injury, turbinate lateralization.[7,8] Levine and Rabago on an examination of adverse events during a post-marketing assessment of balloon sinuplasty identified a total of 3 major complications among 28,500 patients, with a total of >85000 treated sinuses.[8] Balloon sinuplasty although is considered to be a safe technique, in an inexperienced hands or wrongly applied, complications may occur, as with any surgical tool rigid enough to breach through skull base.[7] No serious adverse events or complications were reported between one year and two years in the 65 study patients.[9] If fluoroscopy is used, the risk of radiation exposure should be kept in mind, especially to the lens leading to lenticular opacity (Chandra 2007).

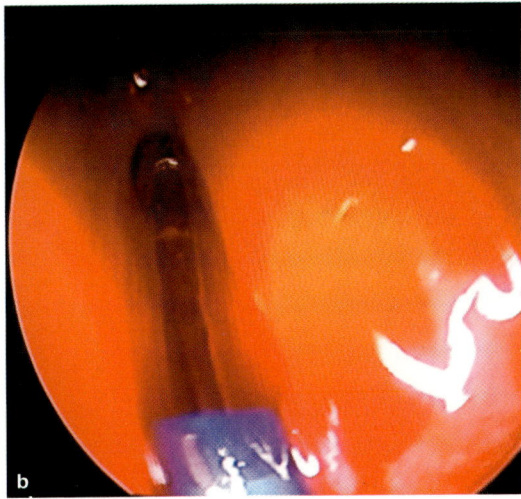

**Fig. 16.4:** (a)Balloon catheter being withdrawn after dilatation, (b) the cannula being passed to irrigate the frontal sinus after dilatation

not require removal and gets absorbed with the course of time. It provides excellent anti-inflammatory action and relieves edema around the ostium.

### Advantages

- Safe and effective.
- Less invasive.
- Minimal bleeding.

## REFERENCES AND FURTHER READING

1. Nayak DR, Balakrishnan R, Murty KD. Endoscopic physiologic approach to allergy-associated chronic rhinosinusitis: a preliminary study. Ear Nose Throat J. 2001, 80:390–403.

2. Brown CL, Bolger WC. Safety and feasibility of balloon catheter dilation of paranasal sinus ostia: a preliminary investigation. Ann Otol Rhino Laryngol. 2006, 115:293–9.

3. Bolger WE, Brown CL, Church CA, Goldberg AN, Karanfilov B, Kuhn FA, et al. Safety and outcomes of balloon catheter sinusotomy: a multicenter 24-week analysis in 115 patients.Otolaryngol Head Neck Surg. 2007, 137:10–20.

4. Brown CL, Bolger WC. Safety and feasibility of balloon catheter dilation of paranasal sinus ostia: a preliminary investigation. Ann Otol Rhino Laryngol. 2006, 115:293–9.

5. Levine HL, Sertich AP 2nd, Hoisington DR, Weiss RL, Pritikin J. Multicenter registry of balloon catheter sinusotomy outcomes for 1,036 patients. Ann Otol Rhinol Laryngol. 2008, 117(4):263–70.

6. Joao Flavio Nogueira Junior, Maria Laura Solferini Silva, Fabio Pires Santos, Aldo Cassol Stamm.; Balloon Sinuplasty: a New Concept in the Endoscopic Nasal Surgery. Intl. Arch. Otorhinolaryngol., São Paulo, 2008; v.12, n.4, pp 538–545.

7. Tomazic PV, Stammberger H, Koele W, Gerstnberer C. Ethmoid roof CSF leak following frontal sinus balloon plasty Rhinology. 2010 June; 48(2):247–50.

8. Howard Levine, and David Rabago, Postgraduate medicine. 2011; 123(2):112–8.

9. Raymond L. Weiss, MD, Christopher A. Church, MD. Frederick A. Kuhn, MD, Howard L. Levine, MD, Michael J. Sillers, MD, and Winston C. Vaughan, MD. Long-term outcome analysis of balloon catheter sinusotomy: Two-year follow-up Otolaryngology—Head and Neck Surgery. 2008; 139, S38–S46.

10. Chandra RK. Estimate of radiation dose to the lens in balloon sinuplasty. Otolaryngol. Head Neck Surg. 2007; 137(6):953–5.

# 17

# Endoscopic Repair of the CSF Rhinorrhea

**Definition:** Leakage of cerebrospinal fluid (CSF) from a fistula between the dura and the skull base leading to discharge of CSF from the nose. Dandy in 1926 was the first person to perform a surgical repair of CSF leak by a frontal craniotomy. Wigand in 1981 used the endoscope to assist the repair of a skull base defect with CSF rhinorrhea. In the last three decades, endoscopic repair has become the preferred method to deal with CSF rhinorrhea.

## ANATOMICAL CLASSIFICATION

- Frontal sinus
- Ethmoid sinus
- Cribriform plate
- Sphenoid sinus
- Paradoxical (eustachian tube)

## Etiology

Can be classified as traumatic or non-traumatic.

## Traumatic

Majority of the cases of CSF rhinorrhea occurs as a result of trauma and the incidence can vary from 80–90%. The commonest sites of CSF leak following trauma are anterior cranial fossa floor (cribriform plate and fovea ethmoidalis) and the posterior wall of the frontal sinus (Iffenecker *et al*. 1999).

- **Non-surgical:** This is the most common cause of CSF rhinorrhea and is usually associated with closed head trauma that may present with an immediate or delayed onset.

- **Surgical:** CSF leak commonly occurs following endoscopic surgery of the nose and paranasal sinus or major skull base surgery involving anterior cranial fossa for tumor removal or inflammatory disease. Although the incidence of CSF leak following endoscopic sinus surgery is less than 2% it is still one of the most common causes of CSF leak (Brodie 1997). This can be present with immediate or delayed onset. The common sites being fovea ethmoidalis and lateral cribriform lamella.

## Non-traumatic

A. **High pressure:** Conditions that increase the ventricular pressure can cause CSF rhinorrhea.
  - **Tumor**
    – Direct infiltration of dura
    – Indirectly due to raised intracranial tension
  - **Hydrocephalus**
B. **Normal pressure**
  - **Congenital:** Spontaneous CSF leak can be associated with congenital bony dehiscence with prolapsed of arachnoid granulations. This can be associated with meningoceles or meningoencephaloceles.
  - **Focal atrophy of the dura** at the cranial defect may lead to CSF leak.
  - **Osteomyelitic erosion**
  - **Idiopathic:** This occurs due to spontaneous rupture of the meningeal dura and fistula formation due to pre-existing

intracranial problem. The term idiopathic although used for unexplained CSF leak, in reality are secondary to raised CSF pressure of varied intracranial causes. Rarely arachnoid granulations along the cribriform plate can cause spontaneous leak.

## CLINICAL FEATURES

Recurrent clear and nonsticky watery fluid draining from nose, often unilateral is the frequent presenting symptom. Any such case of unilateral watery rhinorrhea should be investigated thoroughly and should be suspected for CSF leak unless otherwise proved and should never be treated with steroid nasal spray till the diagnosis is established. Hyposmia/anosmia are associated with 60–80% of cases. Headache is seen in 20% of cases and associated meningitis or raised intracranial pressure should be ruled out. Recurrent meningitis may be associated with CSF leak and will always present with classical features including fever. Wet handkerchief from nasal secretions that fails to dry without stiffening should be suspected for CSF leak (Handkerchief test).

### Investigations

1. **Testing of nasal secretions:**
   a. Beta 2 transferrin assay: It is a highly sensitive test as Beta 2 transferrin is only found in CSF, perilymph and the aqueous humor
   b. Glucose protein determination is a highly unreliable but rapid test
   c. Beta-trace protein is not a very specific test

2. **Diagnostic nasal endoscopy:** It is one of the useful investigations that may help in identifying the site of the leak in certain cases and particularly post-surgical cases but in general has a very limited role in diagnosis of the majority of the cases. Injection of intrathecal fluorescein has been used to diagnose and localize the site(s) of CSF rhinorrhea during nasal endoscopy usually 30 minutes after injection at a dose

of 0.1 mL of 10% non-ophthalmic solution is diluted in 10 mL of CSF and reinjected into the subarachnoid space over a period of 10 minutes. This test can also be done at the time of surgery to facilitate immediate repair.

3. **Imaging studies:**
   a. **HRCT paranasal sinus and the skull base** is the imaging of choice to identify the defect in the skull base with CSF rhinorrhea (Fig. 17.1).
   b. **CT cisternography:** CT scans with or without intrathecal contrast and preoperative nasal endoscopy are the most frequently used investigation to preoperatively localize the site of the leak. Intrathecal contrast injection before the CT scan can provide more accurate information about the leakage (Jones *et al.* 2000).

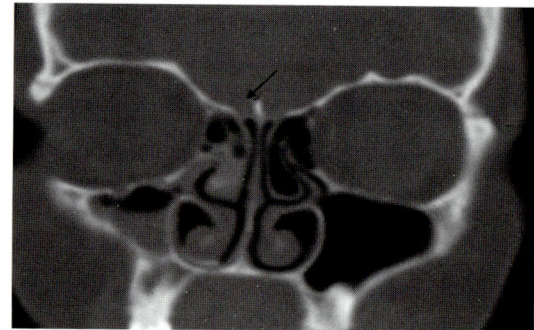

**Fig. 17.1:** CT scan showing the leak site at the attachment of the middle turbinate to fovea ethmoidalis. Also note associated maxillary sinusitis

   c. **Metrizamide CT cisternography:** It is the best tool in establishing the diagnosis and to locate the site of leak
   d. **MRI and MRI cisternography:** Non-invasive images to locate leak site (Fig. 17.2) .

### Management

Most of CSF leaks can close spontaneously within 7 to 10 days with conservative management. The risk of meningitis and other intracranial complications should be kept in

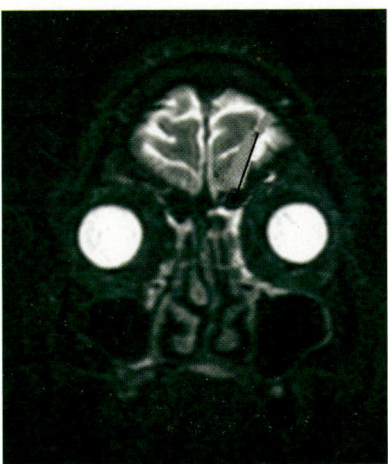

**Fig. 17.2:** MRI showing the leak site in the fovea ethmoidalis (black arrow)

mind in post-traumatic cases and surgical intervention should be the preferred modality apart from antibiotics and other medical treatment.

## Medical Treatment

1. Prophylactic antibiotic.
2. Bed rest in head up position (head of bed position at 15–30°)
3. Coughing, sneezing, and nose blowing, weight lifting needs to be avoided and should be adequately treated whenever present.
4. Mild laxative to prevent increase in CSF pressure.
5. Repeated or continuous lumbar puncture may be requiring in certain cases. The timing for surgery and CSF drainage procedures must be decided with great care and with a clear strategy (22).
6. Diuretics like acetazolamide can be given.
7. Manitol can be started preoperatively.

## SURGICAL TREATMENT

### Basic Principles of Surgery

- Positive identification of leak site
- Meticulous preparation of recipient bed
- Accurate placement of an appropriate graft material

This includes two approaches:

1. **Intracranial:** This approach was frequently being used by a frontal craniotomy approach and still a preferred approach for selected cases by the neurosurgeon. Repair includes the use of pedicled pericranial or dural flap. Some surgeons prefer fascia lata graft for repair.

2. **Extracranial:**

   a. **External or combined endoscopic approach:** Commonly approached with a bi-coronal incision and osteoplastic flap to expose the posterior table of the frontal bone to locate the defect in that area. This approach is particularly suitable for defect above the floor. Graft material like fascia lata and bone/cartilage can be used to seal the defect.

   A combined approach also can be advocated by using a small incision in the eyebrow and frontal sinus trephination for endoscopic visualization and instrument manipulation along with endoscopic frontal sinusotomy.

   b. **Endoscopic approach:**

      i. Overlay Technique
         1. Localize the skull base defect.
         2. Surrounding mucosa is elevated at least 3–5 mm in all direction to prevent mucosa from interfering with graft adhesion.
         3. Place the free graft, which is glued over the underlying structure.

      ii. Underlay Technique
         1. Localize the site of the defect.
         2. Elevate the dura of the skull base for 2–3 mm, thus creating the epidural space.
         3. Connective tissue graft is placed in this pocket.
         4. Then proceed to remove the mucosa as in overlay technique.
         5. Placing the overlay graft.
         6. Thus triple layer seal is achieved.
         7. Useful for large defect.

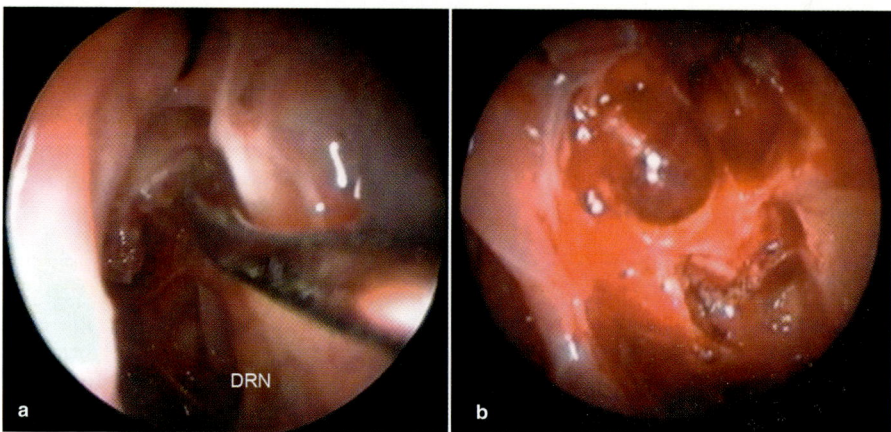

**Fig. 17.3:** (a) The leak site being expose by removing mucosa over the small area of herniated brain tissue, (b) Striping of the mucosa to create a raw bony surface around for graft placement

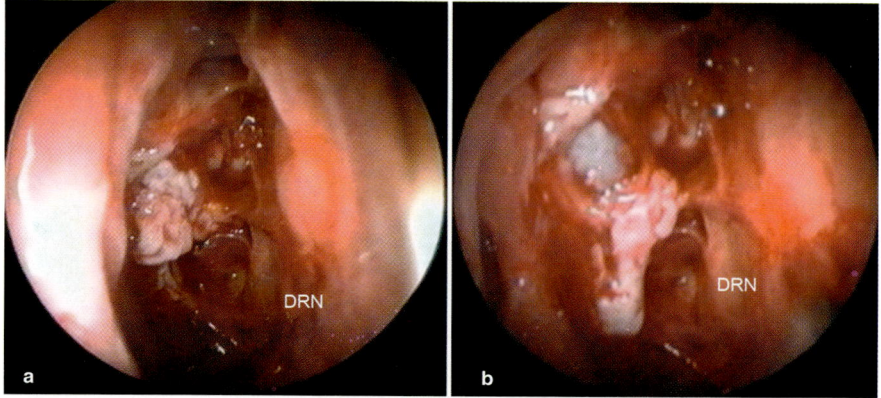

**Fig. 17.4:** (a) Placement of an underlay fascia lata graft followed by placement of a cartilage. Note part of the fascia has been outside to prevent migration of the cartilage

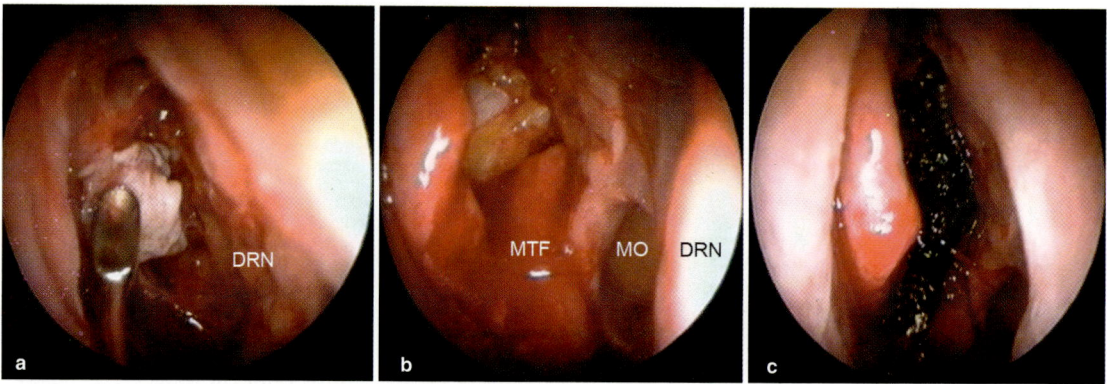

**Fig. 17.5:** (a) Placement of an additional fascia lata,(b) Middle turbinate being partially resected as a pedicled flap (MTF) and placed over graft for early epithelialization and (c) Surgical is placed over the flap to keep it in place

## Indications and Surgical Details

It is one of the most preferred approaches at present with a success rate of more than 90–95% in an experienced hand. Some surgeon prefers to put a lumbar drain prior to surgery to inject intrathecal fluorescein. The key to endoscopic repair is the accurate identification of the site of the leak as well as the relevant anatomy of the area so as to make proper surgical planning. Depending on the site of the leak and the exposure needed, a complete Ethmoidectomy, maxillary and frontal sinusotomy, sphenoidotomy, middle and superior turbinectomies may be required. After identifying the leak, the graft bed is prepared by striping/elevating the surrounding mucosa from the bone (Fig. 17.3a and b). For a small defect Fat graft is preferred to give a dumbbell shaped seal followed by an additional layer of fascia lata as onlay graft. In case of a larger leak with bony defect of more than 1 cm, an underlay bone or cartilage gafting is done in addition to fascial graft placement to prevent prolapsed of brain or meningeal tissue and also to hold the graft in place (Fig. 17.4a and b). If the mucosa is elevated as a flap instead of being striped, it can be reapplied over the graft to facilitate early epithelilization (Fig. 17.5a and b). Alternatively, part of the middle turbinate can be used as a pedicled flap. Application of Surgical® helps in stabilizing the graft in place followed by Merocel (Fig. 17.5c). The first author of this book (DRN) prefers Nasopore® soaked with antibiotic solution for the same as it does not prevent early epithelialization. Immediately after surgery, the surgeon should request the anesthesiologist for removal of the swallowed blood clot from the stomach. Antiemetic is given immediately after surgery before patient is recovered from anaesthesia to prevent postoperative nausea and vomiting.

## Postoperative Treatment

i. Placement of a lumbar drainage
ii. Head end of the bed is elevated to 15–30°
iii. Bed rest
iv. Stool softener
v. Diuretics
vi. Pack removal on 10th day
vii. Light activity after 6 weeks of surgery.

*Postoperative follow-up:* This is absolutely essential as recurrent CSF leak at an alternate site after recent repair is common. Regular endoscopic inspection with minimal debridement of the surgical site should be performed over the long term to identify recurrence of disease.

## REFERENCES AND FURTHER READING

1. Brodie H. Prophylactic Antibiotics for Posttraumatic Cerebrospinal Fluid Fistulae: A Meta-analysis. Archives of Oto: Vol 123(7). July 1997: 749–752.

2. Iffenecker C, Benoudiba F, Parker F, Fuerxer F, David P, Tadie M, et al. The place of MRI in the study of cerebrospinal fluid fistulas. J Radiol 1999; 80:37–43.

3. Jones ME, Reino T, Gnoy A, Guillory S, Wackym P, Lawson W. Identification of intranasal cerebrospinal fluid leaks by topical application with fluorescein dye. Am J Rhinol 2000; 14:93–6.

4. Dandy WD. Pneumocephalus. Arch surg 1926; 12:949–82.

5. Wigand ME Transnasal ethmoidectomy under endoscopic control. Rhinology 1981;19:7–15.

# 18

# The Role of Nasal Endoscopy in Nasopharyngeal Cancer

*Prof. Jaspal Singh Sahota*

## INTRODUCTION

The rigid nasal endoscope, now used by nearly all ENT surgeons, was developed in the 1970s and was instrumental in changing the diagnostic and therapeutic modalities for treatment of sinonasal pathology, especially chronic sinusitis. As surgeons became more experienced in nasal endoscopy, its use expanded to include the diagnosis and treatment of various nasal masses and nasopharyngeal pathology. The use of the nasal endoscope not only permits close, accurate, and magnified views of the nasal cavities and the nasopharynx but also proves immensely useful in diagnosing small submucosal lesions which, otherwise, would be missed by conventional techniques. Traditionally, the nasopharynx is difficult to visualize using speculums since the view is often limited by anatomic and pathologic variations like deviated septum, hypertrophied turbinate, or concha bullosa. Post-nasal examinations using mirrors are also complicated by a limited view and the gag reflex which precludes a thorough examination. The use of the nasal endoscope to evaluate the nasopharynx is, therefore, particularly useful.

## ANATOMY OF THE NASOPHARYNX

The nasopharynx measures about 4 cm high, 4 cm wide, and 3 cm anteroposteriorly. The posterior wall is located about 8 cm from the Pyriform aperture. Endoscopic assessment of the nasopharynx is usually done with the 0° rigid endoscope. The most important region of the nasopharynx with respect to nasopharyngeal cancer is the fossa of Rosenmuller. This recess/region measures up to 2.5 cm in depth and is located between the lateral and posterior walls, just behind the torus. The eustachian tube orifice lies on the lateral wall about 1.5 cm from the roof, posterior wall, choana, and floor.

## Endoscopic Diagnosis of Nasopharyngeal Cancer

Typically, patients with suspected Naso-pharyngeal cancer usually present a hard lymph node swelling just below the angle of the mandible. These patients may also have nasal symptoms and some will have a unilateral hearing loss caused by the obstruction of the eustachian tube either by tumor, edema, or lymphoid enlargement around the tubal orifice. Consequently, the endoscope is used to visualize the region around the fossa of Rosenmuller and the eustachian tube. A suspected lesion may appear as a submucosal bulge, a frank growth, or an infiltrating lesion (Fig. 18.1). There may be edema around the orifice of the eustachian tube endoscopic photograph showing a large tumor arising from the left fossa of Rosenmuller (Fig. 18.2). The eustachian tube opening is seen just interiorly. Indeed, the endoscope has revolutionized the diagnosis of such lesions by enabling the surgeon to take focused, targeted biopsies from this region. Before the advent and use of endoscopes, one had to rely

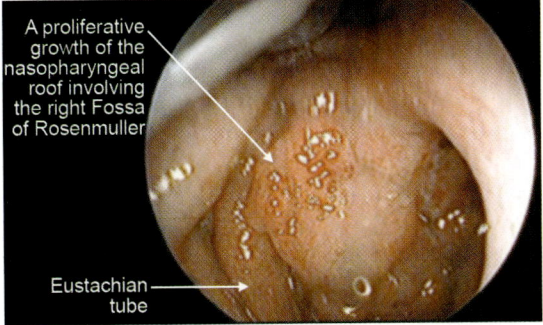

A proliferative growth of the nasopharyngeal roof involving the right Fossa of Rosenmuller

Eustachian tube

**Fig. 18.1:** Proliferative growth of the nasopharynx

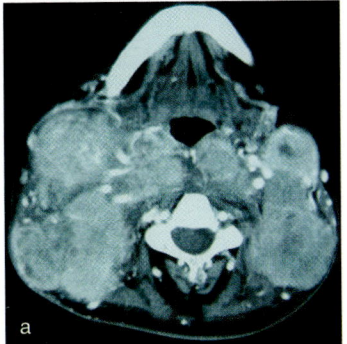

a

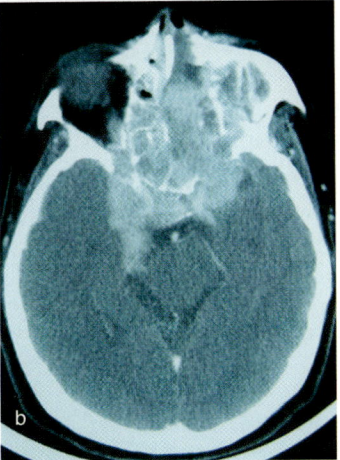

b

on "blind" punch biopsies from the naso-pharynx, which did not always detect small malignant lesions. Now, such biopsies can be taken in the outpatient department and at the same time the rest of the nose and sinuses can be examined.

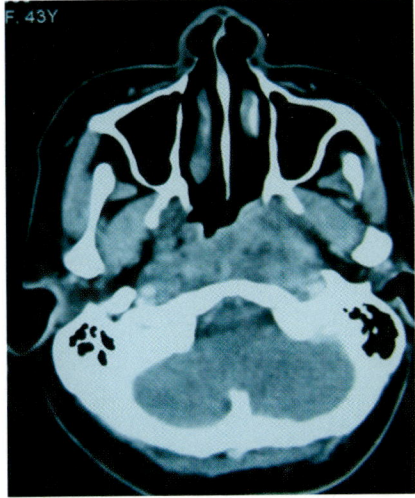

**Fig. 18.2:** Involvement of (L) fossa of Rosenmuller

**Fig. 18.3:** (a) Infiltration into paraphysical space infratemporal fossa with fungating neck nodes, (b) intracranial extension

## Role of Preoperative CT Scan

CT evaluation is very important to detect tumor extension, especially erosion of the bone: contrast CT can show enhancement of the tumor and helps in evaluation of the neck node. Besides nasopharynx, CT of brain and CT neck should be done to rule out intra-cranial involvement and involvement of neck node (Figs 18.3a,b and 18.4).

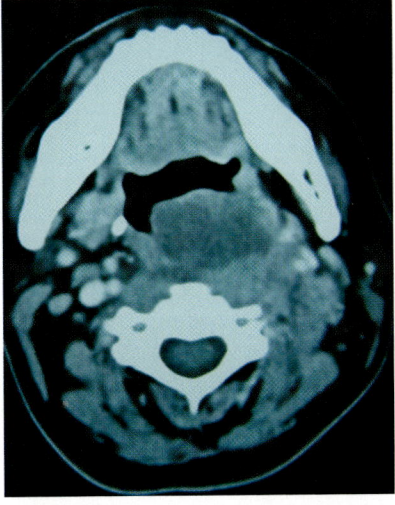

**Fig. 18.4:** Involvement of prevertebral fascia

## Newer Modalities for Diagnosis of NPC

Narrow Band Imaging is fast emerging as an efficient diagnostic and screening modality for early nasopharyngeal cancers. Wang *et al.* report that Narrow band Imaging when used with Nasal Endoscopy is a rapid and effective screening tool for nasopharyngeal cancers. Contact endoscopy using Methylene blue to stain for malignant epithelium was evaluated by Pak et al. 1991. In this method, the suspicious areas are stained with methylene blue and viewed with an endoscope. The malignant epithelium shows distinct patterns when compared with normal epithelium of the nasopharynx.

## The Role of Endoscopes in the Treatment of Nasopharyngeal Cancer

Although most patients will undergo external beam radiotherapy as the standard treatment for their disease, some patients will require salvage therapy in the form of a localized nasopharyngectomy. Accurate mapping of the tumor and its anatomical localization is essential in planning precise radiotherapy because radiotherapy can cause complications like choanal atresia or stenosis. Chronic sinusitis occurs due to blockage of sinus ostia by radiation induced edema. Endoscopic techniques prove to be useful in the aforesaid conditions. Endoscopic nasopharyngectomy for locally recurrent nasopharyngeal carcinoma have been performed with encouraging results (Rohaizam 2009).

## SURGICAL TECHNIQUE

1. After creation of a posteriorly and inferiorly based septal flap (Hadad-Bassagasteguy flap) in the healthy side the posterior half of the bony nasal septum is removed to gain access to the contralateral Rosenmuller fossa.

2. Resection of the posterior half of the nasal septum increases the maneuverability of endoscopes and instruments to facilitate the access.

3. Resection of inferior turbinate's is warranted to provide better access.

4. The curved-blade harmonic scalpel/KTP532 laser is utilized to achieve a bloodless mucosal incision on the nasopharynx, and for a wide resection of tumor.

5. Margins should be taken for histopathological confirmation.

6. First, superior mucosal incision is given followed by the lateral wall, including the cartilaginous portion of the eustachian tube, the roof of the nasopharynx and the inferior margins are resected depending on the extent.

7. Difficulties are usually encountered in peeling the mucosa and periosteum from the bony nasopharynx.

8. The exposed bony surface with flaps is compulsory to prevent infection or osteoradionecrosis in irradiated patients.

9. Hadad rotational flap is used from septum and alternately an inferior turbinate flap can be used and can be glued and packed. Packs are removed after 24–48 hours.

10. Patients can be discharged home within two to three days after the surgery.

## CONCLUSION

Endoscopic evaluation of the nasopharynx is an indispensable tool in the diagnosis and treatment of tumors of the nasopharynx. It permits accurate localization and evaluation and allows targeted biopsies, resulting in improved diagnostic yield. Further advances such as contact endoscopy and narrow band imaging will help in early diagnosis and greatly aid in screening as well.

## REFERENCES AND FURTHER READING

1. Wang *et al.* Nasopharyngeal carcinoma detected by narrow-band imaging endoscopy, Oral Oncol. 2011 Aug; 47(8):736–41. Epub 2011 Mar 9.
2. Pak *et al.* In vivo diagnosis of nasopharyngeal carcinoma using contact rhinoscopy. Laryngoscope. 2001 Aug; 111(8):1453–8.
3. J Rohaizam, Endoscopic Nasopharyngectomy: The Sarawak Experience; Med J Malaysia Vol- 64 No 3 September 2009.

# 19

# Allergic Fungal Rhinosinusitis

Allergic fungal sinusitis (AFS) is a noninvasive form of highly recurrent chronic allergic hypertrophic rhinosinusitis that can be distinguished clinically, histopathologically and prognostically from other forms of chronic fungal rhinosinusitis. It is a form of noninvasive fungal rhinosinusitis and is associated with a hypertrophic sinus disease (HSD). It has clinicopathological features that make it similar, but not identical, to allergic bronchopulmonary aspergillosis (ABPA).

The classification of fungal sinusitis described by deShazo *et al.* (1997) Ferguson (2000) and Adelson et al. (2005) into different invasive and non-invasive types. However, consensus on terminology, pathogenesis, and optimal management is lacking. The International Society for Human and Animal Mycology convened a working group to attempt consensus on the terminology and disease classification has led to the following conclusion (Chakarbati A.; Denning D.; Fergusson B.; Ponikau J. et al. 2009).

## Fungal Rhinosinusitis (FRS)

*Invasive:*
- Acute fulminant invasive fungal sinusitis (AFIFS)
- Chronic invasive fungal sinusitis (CIFS)
- Granulomatous invasive fungal sinusitis (GIFS)

*Non-invasive:*
- Saprophytic fungal infestation (SFI)
- Sinus fungus ball (SFB)

- Fungus-related eosinophilic rhinosinusitis
- Allergic fungal rhinosinusitis (AFRS)
- Eosinofil mucin rhinosinusitis (EMRS)
- Eosinophilic fungal rhinosinusitis (EFRS)

AFS is a recently described clinical entity that has gained increased attention as a cause of chronic sinusitis. Allergic aspergillosis was first recognized by Lamb and Miller 1982 (ABPA). Allergic fungal sinusitis (AFS) was first described by Katzenstein *et al.* (1983), when histopathological similarities were noted between the surgically removed sinus debris of some patients with sinusitis and the bronchial mucus plugs of patients with allergic bronchopulmonary aspergillosis.

The term allergic fungal sinusitis was first coined by Robson *et al.* in 1989. It is the most common type of fungal rhinosinusitis. Allergic bronchopulmonary aspergillosis, a disorder analogous to AFS, was recently reported to have HLA-MHC class II associations.

## Pathogenesis

Allergic fungal sinusitis is mediated by both Type-I (IgE) and Type-III (IgG antigen immune complexes) Gell and Coomb reactions. Patients with allergic fungal sinusitis and hypertrophic sinus disease have HLA-DQB1 03 alleles as a risk factor for disease, with AFS having the highest association. The association of ABPA, AFS, and HSD with class II genes of the major histocompatibility complex places the initiation of these inflammatory diseases within the context of antigen presentation and the acquired immune response.

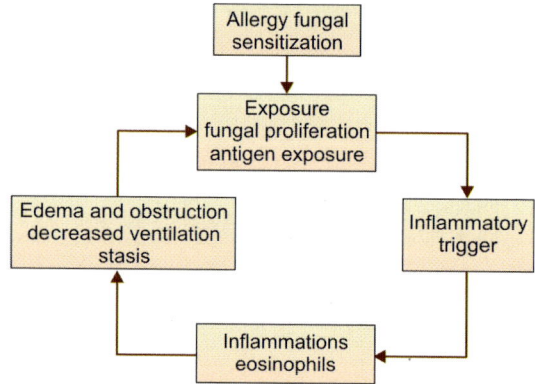

**Fig. 19.1:** The events associated following exposure to fungal antigen

It is a benign noninvasive sinus disease related to a hypersensitivity reaction to fungal antigens that triggers inflammatory response leading to edema and obstruction of the affected sinus ostium and forms a vicious cycle (Fig. 19.1). It should be suspected in any atopic patient with refractory nasal polyps.

## Commom Fungi Involved

- *Aspergillus fumigatus*
- *Bipolaris*
- *Drechslera*
- *Alternaria*
- *Curvularia*
- *Exserohilum*

**Diagnostic criteria:** Bent and Kuhn (1996) proposed diagnostic criteria for allergic fungal sinusitis. This has been divided further into two groups, i.e. major and minor.

### Major Criteria

- Type-I hypersensitivity
- Nasal polyposis
- Characteristic CT findings
- Positive fungal smear
- Allergic mucin with fungal elements and no tissue invasion

### Minor Criteria

- Asthma
- Unilateral predominance

- Radiographic bone erosion
- Positive fungal culture
- Charcot-Leyden crystals
- Serum eosinophil

**Diagnosis of allergic fungal sinusitis:** Significant overlap exists between the clinical, radiological, and immunological features of AFS, invasive fungal disease, and ethmoidal polyposis. A definitive preoperative differentiation of these entities is desirable for diagnosis as it influences the choice of surgical procedure and the perioperative adjunctive medical treatments (Diwakar *et al.* 2003).

- **History:** A history of sinus disease strongly recalcitrant to traditional medical and even surgical therapy aimed largely at bacterial rhinosinusitis. A detail history should be elicited for the following complaints:
  - Sneezing and a runny nose as seen classically in allergic rhinitis.
  - Nasal obstruction
  - Thick and mucopurulent viscid nasal discharge.
  - Headache
  - Postnasal drip
  - Occasional facial pain
  - Cough seen more at night
- **Objective findings:**
  - **Allergic mucin** (Fig. 19.2): Extramucosal allergic mucin (that is also seen grossly at surgery as a characteristic 'peanut-buttery' material)
  - Fungal specific IgE
  - No evidence of invasion
- **Endoscopic mucosal staging system** (Kupferberg, et al. 1996):
  - Stage 0: No mucosal edema or allergic mucin
  - Stage I: Mucosal edema
  - Stage II: Polypoid edema
  - Stage III: Sinus polyps

**Radiological findings:** Sinus computed tomography scans showing chronic rhino-sinusitis (often with the presence of hyper-attenuating sinus contents). Schubert (2000,

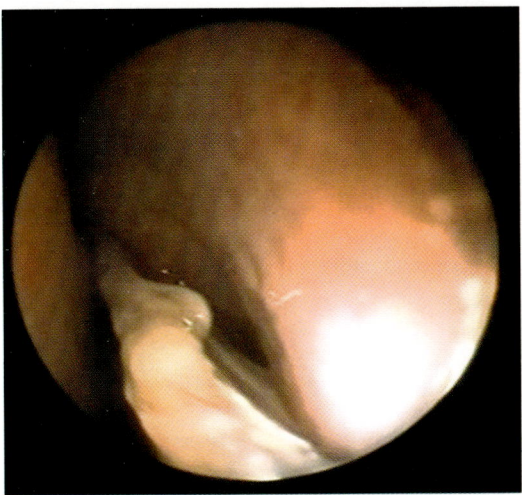

**Fig. 19.2:** Endoscopic picture showing allergic mucin suctioned out from the frontal sinus

2009) noted that computed tomography CT scan are always associated with the abnormal findings in the paranasal sinuses. The characteristic findings that can be noted are:

- Central areas of increased contrast (hyperattenuation) within abnormal paranasal sinuses.
- Marked soft tissue sinus mucosal hyperplasia evident in multiple sinuses.
- Areas of increased density attributed to the presence of fungal-containing allergic mucin.

- Extrasinus extension of the disease is common in the form of expansion.

**Histopathology:** Histopathology shows the presence of eosinophilic-lymphocytic sinus mucosal inflammation and scattered silver stain positive fungal hyphae within the allergic mucin but not in the mucosa. Based on histopathological criteria, Kathleen, et al. (2013) classified fungal sinusitis into following types:

- **Non-invasive FRS**
  - Fungus ball (FB)
  - Allergic fungal rhinosinusitis (AFRS)
  - Mixed FB/AFRS
- **Invasive FRS**
  - Acute (AIFRS)
  - Chronic (CIFRS)
  - Chronic granulomatous (CGFRS)
- **Mixed non-invasive/invasive**
- **Fungal culture:** Fungal cultures should be interpreted with caution. They are best used as supportive evidence because of their variable yield
- **Lab studies:**
  - Elevated total serum IgE
  - Positive inhalant allergy skin tests
  - Microscopically, the mucin often takes on a chondroid appearance with sheets of eosinophils, frequently with the presence of eosinophilic breakdown products or Charcot-Leyden crystals.

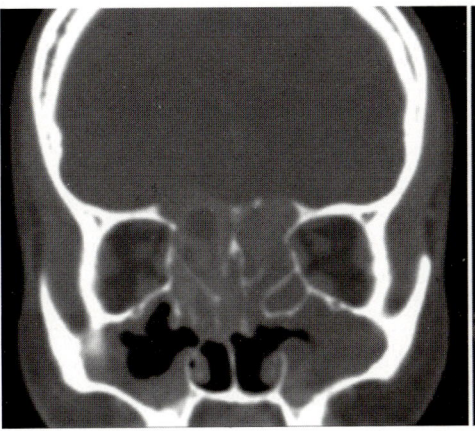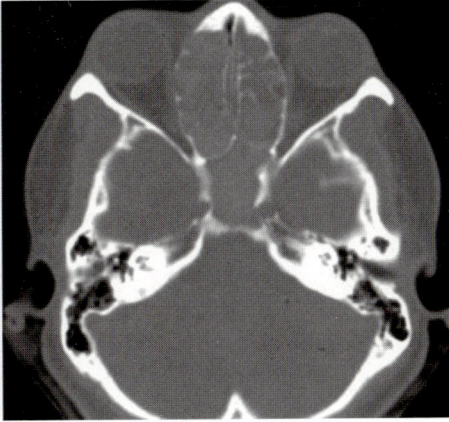

**Fig. 19.3:** (a) Cornal CT, (b) Axial CT, showing hypertrophic sinus diseases associated with areas of hyperattenuation due to fungal containing allergic mucin. Also note expansion of sinus wall

## Treatment

Extensive surgical debridement followed by the use of systemic antifungal agents was initially commonplace. Eventually this notion was challenged by the theory that AFRS represented an immunologic response to presentation of a fungal antigen within a susceptible host (Gungor *et al.* 1998). The initial treatment of extensive allergic fungal sinusitis is surgery to confirm the diagnosis and remove the diseased mucosa (Schubert 1998, 2000). Incomplete surgical removal of the involved hypertrophic sinus tissue may render the patient vulnerable to relapse of allergic fungal sinusitis. Oral corticosteroid therapy post surgery can prevent relapses and potential of corticosteroid side effects needs to be balanced against the risk of recurrent disease.

Surgical treatment involves aggressive sinus surgery followed by aggressive post-operative medical management of allergic inflammatory disease includes allergen immunotherapy, topical and systemic corti-costeroids, antihistamines and antileuko-

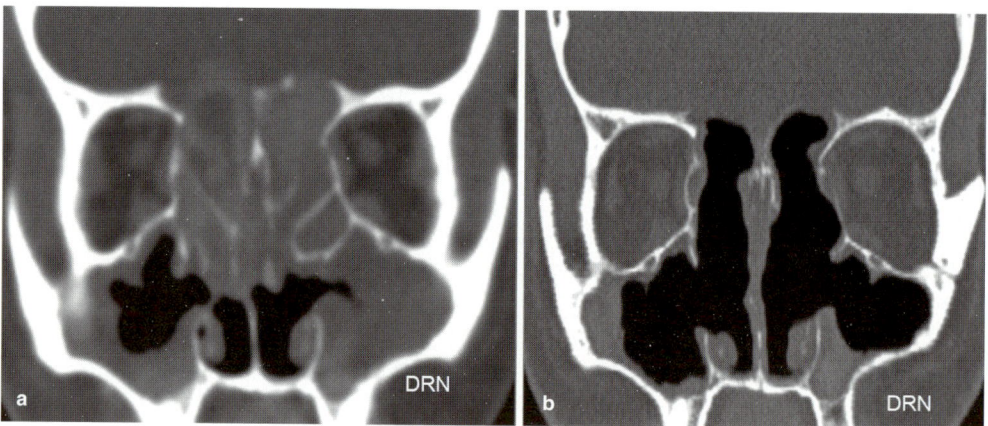

**Fig. 19.4:** (a) Preoperative CT showing allergic fungal sinusitis, (b) Postoperative CT of the same patient showing good clearance of disease

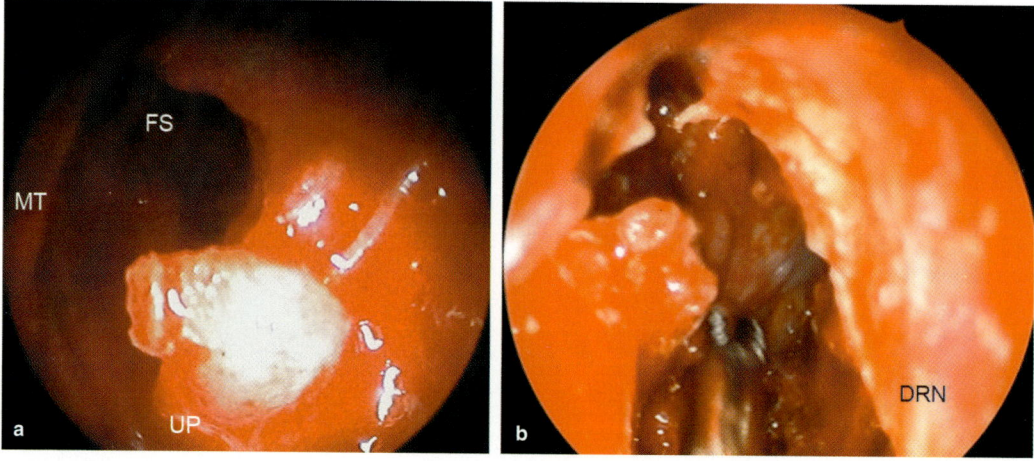

**Fig. 19.5:** (a) Draf type-2 procedure in progress for a case of allergic fungal sinusitis of left frontal sinus, (b) Modified Lothrop procedure for bilateral frontal sinus disease in progress—microdebridor is used to clear the polypoidal tissue

trienes. Radical surgery for AFS has given way to more conservative tissue-sparing appro-aches. Surgery should be conservative but complete, relying almost completely on endoscopic techniques. Treatment of AFS is directed at removal of the inciting antigenic material via complete surgical removal of allergic mucin and debris while also ameliorating the underlying inflammatory process through the use of limited systemic and topical steroid preparations (Mabry 2000).

All patients with AFS should undergo surgical debridement of their sinuses. Extensive disease of the frontal sinus may require a draf (Fig. 19.5a) or a modified Lothrop procedure (Fig. 19.5b). Immunotherapy may be beneficial, rather than harmful, as a component of treatment for AFS. Antifungal therapy often was used in an attempt to provide some degree of control over recurrence of AFS. Data on the effects of this form of therapy for AFS have been limited. Topical application of antifungal agents may hold some benefit in the control of postoperative recurrence. Total serum IgE levels should be followed postoperatively as they can be prognostic for recurrent disease.

Prognosis is good with integrated medical-surgical follow-up, but recurrence remains problematic (Schubert 2006).

## REFERENCES AND FURTHER READING

1. Lamb D, Millar J. Johnston A. Allergic aspergillosis of the paranasal sinuses. J Pathol 1982; 137: 56. 4.
2. Katzenstein A, Sale S, Greenberger P. Pathologic findings in allergic aspergillus sinusitis. J Allergy Clin Immunol 1983; 72:89–93.
3. Schubert et al. Clin Rev Allergy Immunol. 2006 Jun; 30(3):205–16.
4. Bent JP 3rd, Kuhn FA. Antifungal activity against allergic fungal sinusitis organisms. Laryngoscope. 1996 Nov; 106 (11):1331–4.
5. Schubert and Goetz. J Allergy Clin Immunol. 1998; 102:395–402.
6. Gungor et al. Fungal sinusitis: progression of disease in immunosuppression a case report. Ear, Nose and Throat J 1998; 77: 207–215.
7. Schubert M. Ann Allergy Asthma Immunol. (2000) Aug; 85:90–101.
8. Mabry RL, Otolaryngol Head Neck Surg. Jan 2000; 122(1):104–6.
9. Dhiwakar et al. Preoperative Diagnosis of Allergic Fungal Sinusitis. Laryngoscope, (2003) 113: April pp 688–694.
10. Schubert. Clin Rev Allergy Immunol. 2006 Jun; 30(3):205–16.
11. Schubert M. Med Mycol. 2009; 47 Suppl 1:S324–30.
12. deShazo RD et al. Criteria for diagnosing sinus myotome. J allergy clin immunol; 1997,99:475–55.
13. deShazo, et al. Fungal sinusitis N Englant, J Med 1997;337:254–9.
14. Robson M, et al. Aust. NZJ Med. 1989; 19:351–353.
15. Kupferberg SB, Bent JP. Allergic fungal sinusitis in the pediatric population. Archives of Otolaryngology and Head Neck Surgery. 1996;122:1381–84.
16. Ferguson BJ. Definition of fungal rhinosinusitis, Otolaryngology Clinic of North Am 2000;33, 227–35.
17. Chakarbati A, Denning D, Fergusson B, et al. Fungal Rhinosinusitis: A Categorization and Definitional Schema Addressing Current Controversies; Laryngoscope September 2009,119: 1809–18.
18. Kathleen T and Montone et al. Fungal Rhinosinusitis: A Retrospective Microbiologic and Pathologic Review of 400 Patients at a Single University Medical Center, International Journal of Otolaryngology, Vol 2012, Article ID 684835, 9 pages, 2012. doi:10.1155/2012/684835.

# Index